RADIOGRAPHIC POSITIONING
COMPETENCY-BASED APPLICATIONS

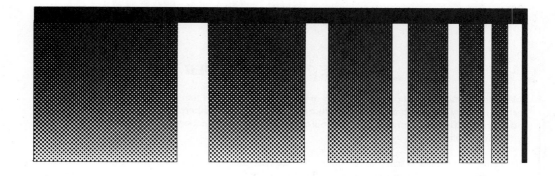

RADIOGRAPHIC POSITIONING
COMPETENCY-BASED APPLICATIONS

James R. Barba, M.A., R.T. (R)
William L. Leonard, M.A., R.T. (R)

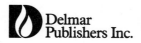 Delmar
Publishers Inc.

NOTICE TO THE READER

Cover design by Kristina Almquist

Delmar Staff
    Executive Editor: David Gordon
    Administrative Editor: Marion Waldman
    Project Editor: Carol Micheli
    Senior Production Supervisor: Larry Main
    Art Supervisor: Judi Orozco
    Design Coordinator: Karen Kemp

For information, address Delmar Publishers Inc.
3 Columbia Circle, Box 15–015
Albany, New York 12203–5015

printed in the United States of America
published simultaneously in Canada
by Nelson Canada,
a division of The Thomson Corporation

1 2 3 4 5 6 7 8 9 10 XXX 99 98 97 96 95 94 93

ISBN: 0-8273-4456-2

CONTENTS

Preface ix

Acknowledgments x

General Positioning Criteria xi

PART 1 Upper Extremity

Fingers (2nd to 5th) 5
Thumb 8
Hand 11
Wrist 14
Forearm 21
Elbow 23
Humerus 33
Shoulder 37
Clavicle 42
Scapula 47
Acromioclavicular Joints 49

PART 2 Lower Extremity

Toes (2nd to 5th) 55
Toe (First) 57
Foot 60
Ankle 64
Calcaneus 67
Tibia and Fibula 73
Knee 75
Femur 89
Hip 92
Pelvis 97

PART 3 Thorax
Chest 103
Ribs 117
Sternum 121
Sternoclavicular Joints 123

PART 4 Abdomen
Abdomen 127

PART 5 Abdomen with Contrast Media
Urinary System 134
Biliary System 144
Gastrointestinal System 152
Barium Enema 166

PART 6 Spinal Column
Cervical Spine 176
Thoracic Spine 184
Lumbosacral Spine 190
Sacrum and Coccyx 198
Sacroiliac Joints 203

PART 7 Cranial and Facial Bones
Skull 213
Optic Foramen 221
Facial Bones 225
Nasal Bones 231
Zygomatic Arches 235
Mandible 239
Temporomandibular Joints 245
Paranasal Sinuses 249
Temporal Bone—Mastoids 255
Temporal Bone—Petrous Portion 261

Bibliography 267

Practice Forms 268

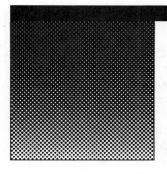

PREFACE

This lab manual is designed as a tool to assist you in achieving the goal of learning radiographic positioning. As part of a learning system, it is one step in the process that will lead you to clinical demonstration and evaluation of your skill as a radiographer.

The manual contains positioning criteria and descriptions for the most common examinations in an outline format. You will be able to use it as your "notebook." The outlined positions will augment your lecture sessions and become your lab notes. You can add information about exposure factors, image criteria, and/or a series of reminder type notes to each page. Blank pages are provided for you to outline additional or special views you will be required to perform for evaluation as part of your clinical education. Patient position drawings are presented to aid your understanding of some of the more complex examinations.

Labeled anatomy drawings are supplied for certain parts of the body. These are standard reference drawings with particular structures labeled. These labeled parts are common areas for study and identification and assist in providing a clear idea of the position of the structure and its general shape. You may use any available sources to review pertinent anatomy. You will review representative radiographs in order to study the end product of your learning.

Additional activities to prepare for the lab session include completing and reviewing the information outlined in lecture, carefully studying anatomy and radiographs of the body part in question, and asking yourself a series of questions such as these:

What is important to observe when evaluating this image for accurate demonstration of anatomy?

What positioning criteria will be utilized to place the patient or part correctly?

How does the movement of the body part or central ray change the relationship of the anatomy lying around the structure(s) of interest?

What similarities or differences can be noted between this new examination and previous examinations studied and practiced?

Once in the lab, you will use the manual to position classmates or radiographic phantoms and to produce and evaluate radiographic images. Identifying and labeling anatomical parts on the radiographs strengthens your ability to analyze your degree of success at positioning and your ability to thoroughly understand how to establish that position. Overall quality of the radiographic image is best evaluated in discussion with your instructor and classmates. Once again, you can use the manual to include notes regarding these activities.

Once you have successfully mastered each position in the lab, you will begin to exercise this newly acquired skill in your clinical course. Familiarize yourself with the radiology department protocols, equipment, exposure factors, and your program's clinical course requirements and clinical evaluation instruments.

The profession of Radiologic Technology has experienced enormous growth in its relatively short life. In addition to the escalated growth in types and technology of imaging equipment, there has been, and will continue to be, an increased emphasis in the educational process of the profession's practitioners. The past ten years have seen radical but necessary modifications in the radiologic technology educational model.

The audience of students and the mobility of the graduates have also undergone a revolution. The average age of student radiographers is on the upswing; and the days of graduates working in the same place, the same modality, and even the same state are gone. The registry has been modified to be clinically or practice oriented.

With this manual, we have attempted to assist both the radiologic technology student and the educator with a practical method to unify the acquisition of the knowledge of radiographic positioning, the keystone of the practice of the profession. We hope it enables each student to look at this knowledge as his or her own and to see the connection between classroom, laboratory, and clinical activities.

TO THE STUDENT

Practice forms are placed together at the back of the book, beginning on p. 268. They are intended to be used in connection with the entire book. These forms may be used to make notes about particular examinations—both those included in this book and others introduced in lectures or lab sessions. You will also use these forms to include examinations specific to your program's clinical site(s).

ACKNOWLEDGMENTS

We would like to express our sincere appreciation to Ms. Sandra Wiskari for her contribution of high quality anatomical and radiographic positioning drawings. We feel that her artistic talents greatly enhanced this manuscript.

We would also like to commend Deborah L. Smith and Mrs. Lee Zukowski for their patience and support in typing the original manuscript.

GENERAL POSITIONING CRITERIA

1. Carefully read the requisition for the type of exam(s) to be performed and the patient's clinical diagnosis and history.
2. Determine the appropriate protocol to be followed for the exam(s) ordered and history and diagnosis recorded.
3. Secure the proper size of image receptors and use proper positioning aids and accessories necessary for the procedure.
4. Greet the patient, stating his or her full name and solicit information to verify his or her identity and the examination to be performed.
5. Check the patient's chart (if available) for pertinent information regarding either history or procedure to be performed.
6. Explain the examination to the patient, including assistance he or she must be able to provide.
7. Assess any variations that may be necessary to the standard positions due to patient condition or trauma.
8. Observe catheters, monitors, chest tubes, oxygen tubings, intravenous or intra-arterial lines and devices, and any other equipment attached to the patient for placement and operation during transfer and while the patient is in your care.
9. Employ universal precautions when coming in contact with blood or other bodily fluids.
10. Utilize appropriate body mechanics when transferring the patient to the x-ray table.
11. Utilize extreme care in handling patients with fractures and trauma patients.
12. Remove any objects that would interfere with or occlude the structure(s) of interest.
13. Secure the patient's valuables.
14. Place the appropriate marker(s) on the image receptors (utilize lead mats if required).
15. Measure the patient and employ gonadal shielding.
16. Set appropriate SID and collimation.
17. Set exposure factors, planning accordingly for seriously injured, geriatric, pediatric, and/or special-needs patients.
18. Position the patient and give clear instructions regarding breathing and maintaining position.
19. While observing the patient, give the instructions, make the exposure, and then inform the patient that he or she may breathe or move.
20. Remove the exposed image receptor, replace with one that is unexposed and position the patient for the next projection.

21. Check SID and collimation and reset the exposure factors.
22. Give clear instructions regarding breathing and maintaining position.
23. Repeat steps 19 through 22 until all projections or examinations have been completed.
24. Process all radiographs and evaluate the quality of all aspects of the resultant images.
25. Follow all departmental protocols regarding the viewing, recording, and disposition of completed radiographs.
26. Give clear postexamination instructions to the patient. These may include diet restrictions, information regarding the availability of the examination's results, etc.
27. Adhere to the departmental protocol for the return of the patient to the proper nursing unit or clinic area.
28. Clean room, restock supplies, and prepare for the next patient.

PART
1

Upper Extremity

Fingers (2nd to 5th) 5

Thumb 8

Hand 11

Wrist 14

Forearm 21

Elbow 23

Humerus 33

Shoulder 37

Clavicle 42

Scapula 47

Acromioclavicular Joints 49

UPPER EXTREMITY

GENERAL TECHNICAL TIPS: DID YOU REMEMBER TO?

■ properly identify the patient?

■ ask a female patient if she may be pregnant?

■ get an accurate history from the patient?

■ determine whether the exam is being performed as the result of trauma or to detect pathology?

■ remove all clothing from the area of interest?

■ remove all jewelry from the area of interest and store it in a safe place?

■ properly shield your patient?

■ check your source-to-image distance?

■ collimate to the part?

■ use a small focal spot whenever possible?

■ utilize appropriate film markers?

■ adjust your original technique when doing post-reduction casted parts?

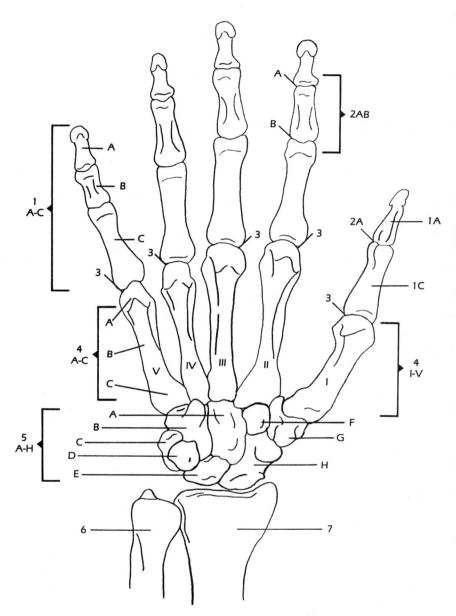

Posterior **A**spect of **H**and and **W**rist

1. Phalanges
  A. Distal
  B. Middle
  C. Proximal
2. Interphalangeal Joints
  A. Distal
  B. Proximal
3. Metacarpophalangeal Joints
4. Metacarpals I–V
  A. Distal End
  B. Shaft
  C. Base

5. Carpals
  A. Capitate—**O**s **M**agnum
  B. Hamate—**U**nciform
  C. Pisiform
  D. Triangular—**T**riquetral
  E. Lunate
  F. Multangular—**T**rapezoid
  G. Greater **M**ultangular—**T**rapezium
  H. Navicular—**S**caphoid
6. Ulna
7. Radius

BODY PART: Fingers (2nd to 5th)

POSITION/PROJECTION: Posteroanterior

ANATOMY: A posteroanterior projection of the carpals, metacarpals, phalanges, the interarticulations of the hand, and the distal ends of the radius and ulna.

PATIENT/PART POSITION: The palmar surface of the hand is placed down on the image receptor with the fingers spread slightly apart.

CENTRAL RAY LOCATION/ANGLE: The central ray is directed perpendicular to the third metacarpophalangeal joint.

NOTES:

BODY PART: Fingers (2nd to 5th)

POSITION/PROJECTION: Oblique

ANATOMY: An oblique projection of the bones and soft tissue of the fingers in question.

PATIENT/PART POSITION: Extending the finger to be examined, rotate the digit 45 degrees from a PA position (2nd and 3rd toward thumb side, 4th and 5th away from thumb). Collimate to the finger being examined.

CENTRAL RAY LOCATION/ANGLE: The central ray is directed perpendicular to the proximal interphalangeal joint.

NOTES:

BODY PART: Fingers (2nd to 5th)

POSITION/PROJECTION: Lateral

ANATOMY: A lateral projection of the phalanges, the distal metacarpals, and the interarticulations of the finger.

PATIENT/PART POSITION: With the finger to be examined extended and the other fingers folded into a fist, the patient's hand should rest either
  a. on the radial surface for the 2nd and 3rd fingers or
  b. on the ulnar surface for the 4th and 5th fingers.

CENTRAL RAY LOCATION/ANGLE: The central ray is directed perpendicular to the proximal interphalangeal joint.

NOTES:

BODY PART: Thumb

POSITION/PROJECTION: Anteroposterior

ANATOMY: An anteroposterior projection of the distal and proximal phalanges of the first metacarpal and its interarticulations.

PATIENT/PART POSITION: The patient will turn his hand into extreme internal rotation, holding back or taping back the 2nd through 5th fingers.

CENTRAL RAY LOCATION/ANGLE: The central ray is directed perpendicular to the first metacarpophalangeal joint.

NOTES:

BODY PART: Thumb

POSITION/PROJECTION: Oblique

ANATOMY: The first finger in an oblique projection (including all bony and soft tissue structures).

PATIENT/PART POSITION: Abduct the thumb and place the palmar surface of the hand on the film.

CENTRAL RAY LOCATION/ANGLE: The central ray is directed perpendicular to the interphalangeal joint of the first finger.

NOTES:

BODY PART: Thumb

POSITION/PROJECTION: Lateral

ANATOMY: The first finger in a lateral projection (including all bony and soft tissue structures).

PATIENT/PART POSITION: Have the patient make a fist with the thumb abducted, then rotate the hand so that the thumb is in a true lateral position.

CENTRAL RAY LOCATION/ANGLE: The central ray is directed perpendicular to the first metacarpophalangeal joint.

NOTES:

BODY PART: Hand

POSITION/PROJECTION: Posteroanterior

ANATOMY: A posteroanterior projection of the carpals, the metacarpals, the phalanges, the interarticulations of the hand, and the distal ends of the radius and ulna.

PATIENT/PART POSITION: The palmar surface of the hand is placed down on the image receptor with the fingers spread slightly apart.

CENTRAL RAY LOCATION/ANGLE: The central ray is directed perpendicular to the third metacarpophalangeal joint and centered to the image receptor.

NOTES:

BODY PART: Hand

POSITION/PROJECTION: Oblique

ANATOMY: An oblique projection of the carpals, metacarpals, phalanges, the interarticulations of the hand, and the distal ends of the radius and ulna.

PATIENT/PART POSITION: With the hand resting palmar surface down, rotate the hand laterally until the hand forms a 45-degree angle with the image receptor. The fingers are slightly flexed so that their tips will touch the image receptor.

CENTRAL RAY LOCATION/ANGLE: The central ray is directed perpendicular to the third metacarpophalangeal joint and centered to the image receptor.

NOTES:

BODY PART: Hand

POSITION/PROJECTION: Lateral—Extension, Flexion

ANATOMY: Hand and wrist should be seen in true lateral projection, with phalanges, metacarpals, carpals, and distal radius and ulna superimposed. The thumb should be seen without superimposition. If performed with the hand in flexion, this projection will demonstrate anterior or posterior displacement in cases of metacarpal fracture(s).

PATIENT/PART POSITION: With the forearm and hand resting on the ulnar surface, the patient will extend the fingers with the thumb 90 degrees to the palm. To place the hand in flexion, place the arm in the same position but have the patient relax the fingers so that the arch of the hand is maintained and the fingers are superimposed. The thumb will still be visualized without superimposition.

CENTRAL RAY LOCATION/ANGLE: The central ray is directed perpendicular to the metacarpophalangeal joints.

NOTES:

The lateral in flexion is a good projection for demonstration of anterior or posterior displacement of metacarpals in trauma cases.

BODY PART: Wrist

POSITION/PROJECTION: Posteroanterior

ANATOMY: A posteroanterior projection of the carpals, the distal ends of the radius and ulna, and the proximal ends of the metacarpals.

PATIENT/PART POSITION: The patient's forearm should rest on the table with the hand and forearm parallel to the image receptor. Arch (cup) the hand by flexing the fingers at the middle phalangeal joints to place the carpals in contact with the image receptor.

CENTRAL RAY LOCATION/ANGLE: The central ray is directed perpendicular to the midcarpal area.

NOTES:

BODY PART: Wrist

POSITION/PROJECTION: Posteroanterior Oblique

ANATOMY: An oblique projection of the carpals on the lateral side of the wrist, especially the navicular.

PATIENT/PART POSITION: With the wrist in the posteroanterior position, rotate the wrist laterally until it forms a 45-degree angle with the image receptor.

CENTRAL RAY LOCATION/ANGLE: The central ray is directed perpendicular to enter at the distal radius.

NOTES:

BODY PART: Wrist

POSITION/PROJECTION: Lateral

ANATOMY: A lateral projection of the carpals, the proximal ends of the metacarpals, and the distal ends of the radius and ulna.

PATIENT/PART POSITION: With the elbow flexed 90 degrees, the patient's arm rests on the ulnar surface. Adjust the forearm and hand so that the wrist is in a true lateral.

CENTRAL RAY LOCATION/ANGLE: The central ray is directed perpendicular to the wrist joint.

NOTES:

BODY PART: Wrist—Special Examinations

POSITION/PROJECTION: Scaphoid—Stecher Method

ANATOMY: The navicular bone, free of superimposition from the surrounding carpals.

PATIENT/PART POSITION: The patient's hand rests in a PA position, on the image receptor, which has been elevated on a 20-degree angle sponge. The elevated end of the cassette is placed at the distal end of the hand. The patient is then placed in ulnar flexion and the carpus centered approximately ½ inch above the midpoint of the cassette.

CENTRAL RAY LOCATION/ANGLE: The central ray is directed perpendicular to the navicular. **Note:** This procedure may also be accomplished by using a 20-degree tube tilt (toward the elbow), with the cassette and wrist horizontal.

NOTES:

BODY PART: Wrist—Special Examinations

POSITION/PROJECTION: Carpal Tunnel—Gaynor-Hart Method

ANATOMY: A tangential projection of the carpal canal, including the palmar aspects of the greater multangular, the tuberosity of the navicular, the lesser multangular, the capitate, the hamular process of the hamate, the triquetrum, and the entire pisiform.

PATIENT/PART POSITION: Hyperextend the wrist and center the image receptor to level of the radial styloid. The long axis of the hand should be perpendicular to the film. Rotate the hand slightly toward the radial side.

CENTRAL RAY LOCATION/ANGLE: The central ray is directed 25 to 30 degrees cephalic to enter approximately 1 inch distal to the base of the fourth metacarpal.

NOTES:

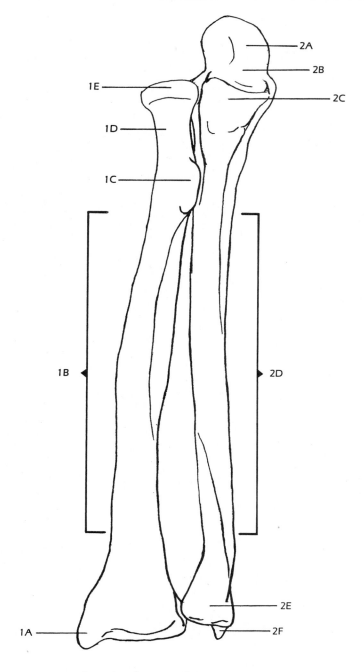

Anterior **A**spect of **R**adius and **U**lna

1. **R**adius
  A. **S**tyloid Process
  B. **S**haft
  C. **R**adial **T**uberosity
  D. **N**eck
  E. **H**ead

2. **U**lna
  A. **O**lecranon **P**rocess
  B. **S**emilunar **N**otch
  C. **C**oronoid **P**rocess
  D. **S**haft
  E. **H**ead
  F. **S**tyloid **P**rocess

BODY PART: Forearm

POSITION/PROJECTION: Anteroposterior

ANATOMY: An anteroposterior projection of the radius, ulna, distal humerus, and proximal row of carpal bones.

PATIENT/PART POSITION: The hand is supinated, the elbow is extended, and the forearm is centered to the unmasked half of the film or across the diagonal axis of the film.

CENTRAL RAY LOCATION/ANGLE: The central ray is directed perpendicular to the midpoint of the forearm.

NOTES:

BODY PART: Forearm

POSITION/PROJECTION: Lateral

ANATOMY: A lateral projection of the radius, ulna, distal humerus, and the proximal row of carpal bones.

PATIENT/PART POSITION: The patient's shoulder should be positioned so that the humerus and shoulder are parallel to the table along with the forearm. The elbow is flexed 90 degrees, and the hand, wrist, and forearm rotated to lie in a true lateral position resting on the ulnar surface.

CENTRAL RAY LOCATION/ANGLE: The central ray is directed perpendicular to the midpoint of the forearm.

NOTES:

BODY PART: Elbow

POSITION/PROJECTION: Anteroposterior

ANATOMY: An anteroposterior projection of the elbow joint, the distal end of the humerus, and the proximal end of the radius and ulna.

PATIENT/PART POSITION: Have the patient supinate the hand and extend the elbow. The hand must be supinated to prevent rotation of the radius and ulna. Center the image receptor to the elbow joint.

CENTRAL RAY LOCATION/ANGLE: The central ray is directed perpendicular to the elbow joint.

NOTES:

BODY PART: Elbow—Special Examinations

POSITION/PROJECTION: Anteroposterior—Acute Flexion

ANATOMY: An anteroposterior projection of the distal humerus and the proximal radius and ulna in two separate exposures.

PATIENT/PART POSITION: Distal humerus: Place the humerus parallel to the image receptor, centering slightly superior to the epicondyloid area. Proximal radius and ulna: Place the humerus parallel to the image receptor, centering two inches superior to the epicondyloid area.

CENTRAL RAY LOCATION/ANGLE: Distal humerus: The central ray is directed perpendicularly to the midpoint of the image receptor. Proximal radius and ulna: The central ray is angled so that it is perpendicular to the forearm and directed to the midpoint of the image receptor.

NOTES:

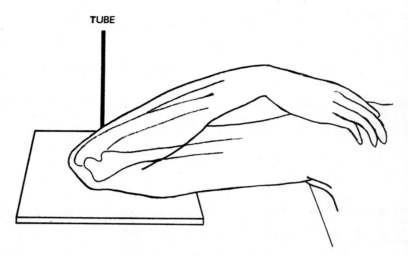

TUBE

Distal Humerus

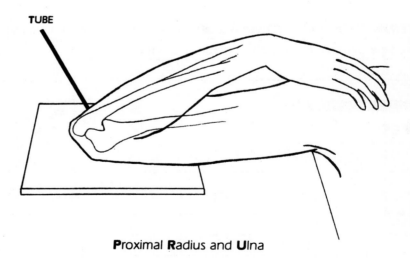

TUBE

Proximal Radius and Ulna

ELBOW—Acute Flexion Position

BODY PART: Elbow—Special Examinations

POSITION/PROJECTION: Anteroposterior—Partial Flexion

ANATOMY: An anteroposterior projection of the distal humerus and the proximal radius and ulna in two separate exposures.

PATIENT/PART POSITION: Distal humerus: Place the humerus parallel to the image receptor, centering the condyloid area of the humerus. It may be necessary to provide support for the patient's forearm. Proximal radius and ulna: Place the dorsal surface of the forearm on the image receptor, centering to the elbow joint.

CENTRAL RAY LOCATION/ANGLE: For either position, the central ray is directed perpendicular to the midpoint of the image receptor.

NOTES:

BODY PART: Elbow

POSITION/PROJECTION: Medial Oblique

ANATOMY: An internal (medial) oblique projection of the elbow joint, distal humerus, and the proximal forearm (radius and ulna). The coronoid process of the ulna is well demonstrated.

PATIENT/PART POSITION: Have the patient pronate the hand and extend the elbow. Center the image receptor to the midpoint of the elbow joint. The anterior surface of the elbow should form a 40- to 45-degree angle with the cassette.

CENTRAL RAY LOCATION/ANGLE: The central ray is directed perpendicular to the midpoint of the elbow joint.

NOTES:

BODY PART: Elbow

POSITION/PROJECTION: Lateral Oblique

ANATOMY: An external (lateral) oblique image of the elbow. The radial head is demonstrated clearly.

PATIENT/PART POSITION: Extend the elbow and center the image receptor to the midpoint of the elbow joint. Externally rotate the hand and arm to place the posterior surface of the elbow at an angle of 40 degrees with the plane of the film.

CENTRAL RAY LOCATION/ANGLE: The central ray is directed perpendicular to the midpoint of the elbow joint.

NOTES:

BODY PART: Elbow

POSITION/PROJECTION: Lateral

ANATOMY: The distal humerus, proximal forearm, and olecranon process. Fat pads should be visualized.

PATIENT/PART POSITION: The patient is seated with the elbow flexed 90 degrees. The shoulder is dropped in order to maintain a parallel relationship between the plane of the image receptor and the humerus and forearm. This should place the condyles of the humerus perpendicular to the image receptor.

CENTRAL RAY LOCATION/ANGLE: The central ray is directed perpendicular to the midpoint of the elbow joint.

NOTES:

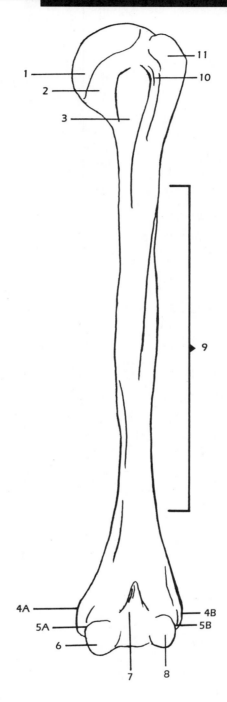

Anterior **A**spect of the **H**umerus

1. **H**ead
2. **A**natomical **N**eck
3. **S**urgical **N**eck
4. **E**picondyle
   A. **M**edial
   B. **L**ateral

5. **C**ondyle
   A. **M**edial
   B. **L**ateral
6. **T**rochlea
7. **C**oronoid **F**ossa

8. **C**apitulum
9. **S**haft
10. **L**esser **T**uberosity
11. **G**reater **T**uberosity

BODY PART: Humerus

POSITION/PROJECTION: Anteroposterior

ANATOMY: An anteroposterior projection of the entire humerus including both the elbow and shoulder joints.

PATIENT/PART POSITION: The image receptor should be placed so that the upper border of the film is 1½ inches above the head of the humerus. Place the arm to be examined in an anatomical anteroposterior position. The desired position will find a coronal plane passing through the epicondyles parallel with the plane of the image receptor.

CENTRAL RAY LOCATION/ANGLE: The central ray is directed perpendicular to the mid-shaft of the humerus.

NOTES:

BODY PART: Humerus

POSITION/PROJECTION: Transthoracic Lateral—Lawrence Method

ANATOMY: A lateral projection of the upper half or two-thirds of the humerus projected through the thorax.

PATIENT/PART POSITION: With the patient seated or standing, the affected side is placed against the upright Bucky. Have the patient elevate the uninjured arm over the head. This will elevate the uninjured shoulder and lower the injured shoulder. Center the image receptor to the region of the surgical neck of the affected side.

CENTRAL RAY LOCATION/ANGLE: Direct the central ray perpendicular to the center of the image receptor.

NOTES:

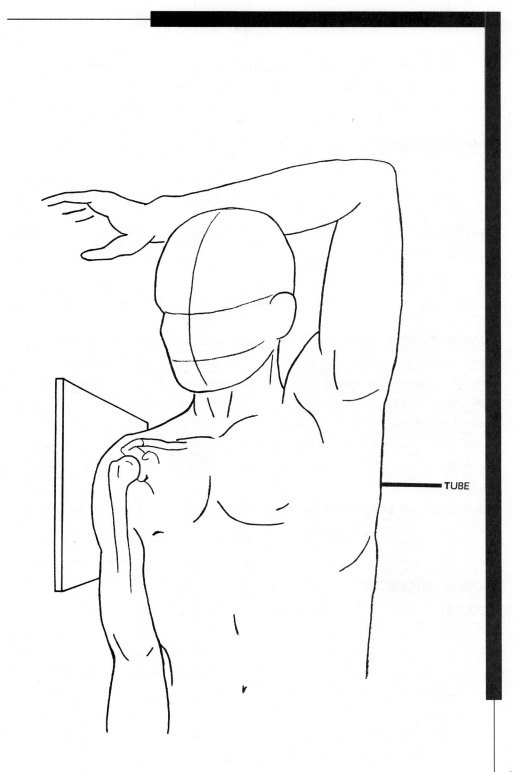

TUBE

Upper **H**umerus
Transthoracic **L**ateral **P**osition

BODY PART: Humerus

POSITION/PROJECTION: Lateral

ANATOMY: A lateral projection of the entire humerus including both the shoulder and elbow joints.

PATIENT/PART POSITION: The image receptor should be placed so that the upper margin of the film is 1½ inches above the head of the humerus. Flex the elbow 90 degrees and rest the forearm across the abdomen. The true lateral will find a coronal plane passing through the epicondyles forming a right angle to the plane of the image receptor. In case of suspected fracture, rotation of the humerus for the lateral will not be possible. It is therefore necessary to do a cross-table lateral of the lower humerus and the transthoracic lateral for the upper humerus.

CENTRAL RAY LOCATION/ANGLE: The central ray is directed perpendicular to the mid-shaft of the humerus.

NOTES:

BODY PART: Shoulder

POSITION/PROJECTION: Anteroposterior—Neutral Rotation

ANATOMY: The posterior part of the supraspinatus insertion site, sometimes profiling small calcific deposits.

PATIENT/PART POSITION: Center the image receptor to the coracoid process and ask the patient to rest the palm against the thigh. This position will place the epicondyles of the elbow at a 45-degree angle to the plane of the film.

CENTRAL RAY LOCATION/ANGLE: The central ray is directed perpendicular to the coracoid process.

NOTES:

BODY PART: Shoulder

POSITION/PROJECTION: Anteroposterior—External Rotation

ANATOMY: The bony and soft tissue structures of the shoulder and proximal humerus, especially the glenohumeral joint, the region of the subacromial bursa, and a profile of the greater tuberosity.

PATIENT/PART POSITION: With the film centered to the coracoid process, ask the patient to turn the palm of the hand forward (supinate the hand) and to abduct the arm slightly so that the coronal plane of the epicondyles is parallel with the plane of the image receptor.

CENTRAL RAY LOCATION/ANGLE: The central ray is directed perpendicular to the coracoid process.

NOTES:

BODY PART: Shoulder

POSITION/PROJECTION: Anteroposterior—Internal Rotation

ANATOMY: The region of the subdeltoid bursa and a profile projection of the site of insertion of the subscapularis tendon.

PATIENT/PART POSITION: With the image receptor centered to the coracoid process, ask the patient to rotate the arm internally, slightly flexing the elbow, until the back of the hand is resting on the hip (the epicondyles are perpendicular to the plane of the film).

CENTRAL RAY LOCATION/ANGLE: The central ray is directed perpendicular to the coracoid process.

NOTES:

BODY PART: Shoulder

POSITION/PROJECTION: Transaxillary Lateral—Lawrence Method

ANATOMY: The glenohumeral joint, the lateral portion of the coracoid process, and the acromioclavicular joint.

PATIENT/PART POSITION: The patient is supine with the affected arm abducted to form a 90-degree angle with the body. Build up the shoulder approximately 3 to 4 inches using a small sponge. Have the patient turn the head away from the side being examined. Place the image receptor as close as possible to the patient's neck.

CENTRAL RAY LOCATION/ANGLE: Direct the central ray horizontally through the axilla to the region of the acromioclavicular articulation. This requires that the tube be angulated medially. The degree of angulation will depend on the degree of abduction of the patient's arm.

NOTES:

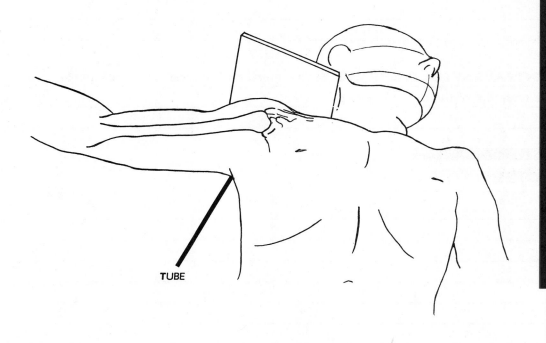

TUBE

Shoulder **J**oint
Transaxillary **L**ateral

BODY PART: Clavicle

POSITION/PROJECTION: Anteroposterior

ANATOMY: An anteroposterior projection of the clavicle. A posteroanterior projection would demonstrate better detail because of decreased object-image distance, but the AP position is used to prevent further displacement in case of fracture.

PATIENT/PART POSITION: Center the image receptor to the point midway between the midsagittal plane of the body and the outer border of the shoulder at the level of the coracoid process.

CENTRAL RAY LOCATION/ANGLE: The central ray is directed perpendicular to the midpoint of the image receptor.

NOTES:

BODY PART: Clavicle

POSITION/PROJECTION: Anteroposterior Axial

ANATOMY: The clavicle, free of superimposition by the ribs.

PATIENT/PART POSITION: The patient is supine or in erect AP position and positioned the same as the AP projection.

CENTRAL RAY LOCATION/ANGLE: Direct the central ray to the supraclavicular fossa at an angle of between 25 and 30 degrees cephalad.

NOTES:

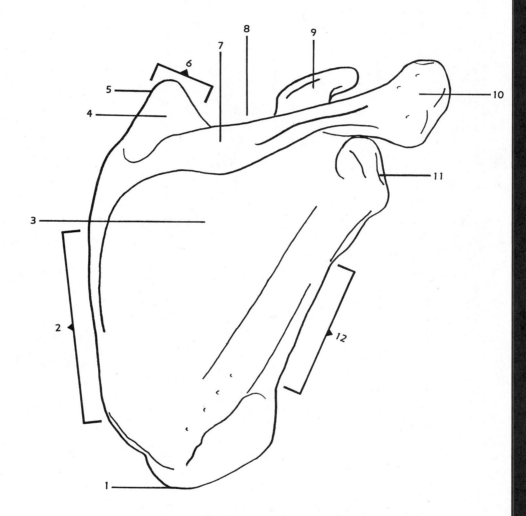

Posterior **A**spect of **S**capula

1. Inferior Angle
2. Vertebral Border
3. Infraspinatus Fossa
4. Supraspinatus Fossa
5. Medial Angle
6. Superior Border

7. Spine
8. Scapular Notch
9. Coracoid Process
10. Acromion
11. Glenoid Fossa
12. Axillary Border

BODY PART: Scapula

POSITION/PROJECTION: Anteroposterior

ANATOMY: The scapula in the anteroposterior projection with the lateral border of the body free of any superimposition.

PATIENT/PART POSITION: Abduct the arm until it forms a 90-degree angle with the body. Center the affected scapula to the midline of the grid or table.

CENTRAL RAY LOCATION/ANGLE: The central ray is directed perpendicular to the midscapular region approximately 2 inches below the coracoid process.

NOTES:

BODY PART: Scapula

POSITION/PROJECTION: Lateral

ANATOMY: The scapula in the lateral projection.

PATIENT/PART POSITION: Direct the patient to face a vertical grid device and reach across the chest to rest the hand of the affected extremity on the shoulder on the unaffected side. Place the image receptor 2 inches above the top of the shoulder. Place the patient in an oblique position with the affected side closest to the vertical grid device. Rotate the patient until the vertebral and axillary borders of the scapula are superimposed.

CENTRAL RAY LOCATION/ANGLE: Direct the central ray perpendicular to the midvertebral border of the scapula.

NOTES:

BODY PART: Acromioclavicular Joints

POSITION/PROJECTION: Anteroposterior—Pearson Method

ANATOMY: A bilateral frontal projection of the acromioclavicular joints. Dislocation, separation, and function of the joints will be seen.

PATIENT/PART POSITION: The patient must be in the erect position either standing or seated with the back against the upright Bucky. Center the midsagittal plane of the body to the center of the image receptor and have the arms hanging at the side. On the first image receptor, an exposure is made with the patient bearing no weight. On the second image receptor, an exposure is made with the patient holding equal weights in each hand.

CENTRAL RAY LOCATION/ANGLE: The central ray is perpendicular to the image receptor, centered to the midline of the body at the level of the AC joints at a 72-inch SID.

NOTES:

PART

2

Lower Extremity

Toes (2nd to 5th) 55

Toe (First) 57

Foot 60

Ankle 64

Calcaneus 67

Tibia and Fibula 73

Knee 75

Femur 89

Hip 92

Pelvis 97

LOWER EXTREMITY

GENERAL TECHNICAL TIPS:
DID YOU
REMEMBER TO?

■ properly identify the patient?

■ ask a female patient if she may be pregnant?

■ get an accurate history from the patient?

■ determine whether the exam is being performed as the result of trauma or to detect pathology?

■ remove all clothing from the area of interest?

■ utilize sheets to repect the patient's modesty when examining the lower extremity?

■ properly shield your patient?

■ check your source-to-image distance?

■ collimate to the part?

■ use a small focal spot whenever possible?

■ utilize appropriate film markers?

■ adjust your original technique when doing post-reduction casted parts?

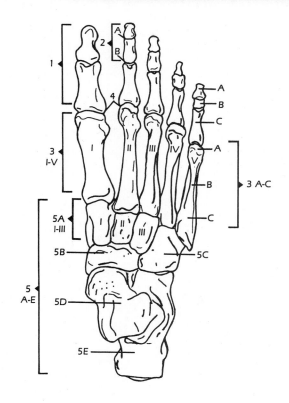

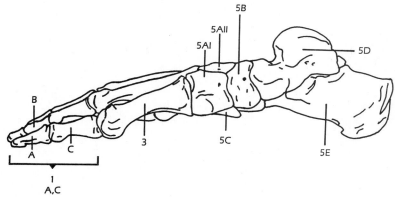

Anterior and **L**ateral **A**spects of **F**oot and **A**nkle

1. **P**halanges
   A. **D**istal
   B. **M**iddle
   C. **P**roximal
2. **I**nterphalangeal **J**oints
   A. **D**istal
   B. **P**roximal
3. **M**etatarsals I–V
   A. **D**istal End
   B. **S**haft
   C. **B**ase

4. **M**etatarsophalangeal **J**oints
5. **T**arsals
   A. **C**uneiforms I, II, III
   B. **N**avicular
   C. **C**uboid
   D. **T**alus
   E. **C**alcaneus

BODY PART: Toes (2nd to 5th)

POSITION/PROJECTION: Anteroposterior of the Foot (Dorsoplantar)

ANATOMY: The tarsals anterior to the talus, the metatarsals, and the phalanges.

PATIENT/PART POSITION: With the plantar surface resting on the film, adjust the foot so that its long axis is parallel to the midline of the image receptor.

CENTRAL RAY LOCATION/ANGLE: The central ray is directed perpendicular to the base of the third metatarsal.

NOTES:

BODY PART: Toes (2nd to 5th)

POSITION/PROJECTION: Medial Oblique

ANATOMY: An oblique projection of the phalanges and the distal metatarsals.

PATIENT/PART POSITION: With the sole of the foot resting on the image receptor, rotate the foot medially so that the plantar surface forms a 30-degree angle with the plane of the image receptor.

CENTRAL RAY LOCATION/ANGLE: The central ray is directed perpendicular to the third metatarsophalangeal joint.

NOTES:

BODY PART: Toe (First)

POSITION/PROJECTION: Anteroposterior of the Foot (Dorsoplantar)

ANATOMY: The tarsals anterior to the talus, the metatarsals, and the phalanges in an anteroposterior projection.

PATIENT/PART POSITION: With the plantar surface resting on the image receptor, adjust the foot so the long axis is parallel to the midline of the image receptor.

CENTRAL RAY LOCATION/ANGLE: The central ray is directed perpendicular to the base of the third metatarsal.

NOTES:

BODY PART: Toe (First)

POSITION/PROJECTION: Medial Oblique

ANATOMY: An oblique projection of the phalanges and the distal metatarsal of the first toe.

PATIENT/PART POSITION: With the plantar surface resting on the image receptor, rotate the foot medially so that the plantar surface forms a 30- to 45-degree angle with the plane of the image receptor.

CENTRAL RAY LOCATION/ANGLE: The central ray is directed perpendicular to the first metatarsophalangeal joint.

NOTES:

BODY PART: Toe (First)

POSITION/PROJECTION: Lateral

ANATOMY: A lateral projection of the phalanges and the distal metatarsal of the first toe.

PATIENT/PART POSITION: With the foot resting on the medial surface, tape the other toes back to prevent superimposition.

CENTRAL RAY LOCATION/ANGLE: The central ray is directed perpendicular to the interphalangeal joint of the first toe.

NOTES:

BODY PART: Foot

POSITION/PROJECTION: Anteroposterior (Dorsoplantar)

ANATOMY: The tarsals anterior to the talus, the metatarsals, and the phalanges.

PATIENT/PART POSITION: With the knee flexed, place the plantar surface of the foot on the image receptor. Adjust the foot so that its long axis is parallel to the midline of the image receptor.

CENTRAL RAY LOCATION/ANGLE: The central ray is directed 10 degrees cephalic and enters at the base of the third metatarsal.

NOTES:

BODY PART: Foot

POSITION/PROJECTION: Medial Oblique

ANATOMY: The interspaces between the cuboid and calcaneus, between the cuboid and the fourth and fifth metatarsals, and between the talus and navicular.

PATIENT/PART POSITION: With the patient's knee flexed, place the plantar surface of the foot on the image receptor. Rotate the foot medially so that the plantar surface forms a 30-degree angle with the surface of the image receptor. Center the image receptor to the level of the base of the fifth metatarsal.

CENTRAL RAY LOCATION/ANGLE: The central ray is directed perpendicular to the midline of the foot at the level of the base of the third metatarsal.

NOTES:

BODY PART: Foot

POSITION/PROJECTION: Lateral

ANATOMY: A lateral projection of the bones (tarsals, metatarsals, and phalanges) and soft tissue of the foot.

PATIENT/PART POSITION: Have the patient roll up toward the affected side. Both the leg and foot should be in the lateral position. The foot should be dorsiflexed and the plantar surface perpendicular to the image receptor.

CENTRAL RAY LOCATION/ANGLE: The central ray is directed perpendicular to the bases of the metatarsals.

NOTES:

BODY PART: Foot—Special Examinations

POSITION/PROJECTION: Lateral Weight-Bearing Feet

ANATOMY: A lateral of the phalanges, metatarsals, and tarsals in a lateral weight-bearing position. It is used to demonstrate the longitudinal arch. Both feet are examined for comparison.

PATIENT/PART POSITION: The patient stands erect in a natural position on a low bench on blocks designed for lateral weight-bearing feet.

CENTRAL RAY LOCATION/ANGLE: The central ray is directed perpendicular to the area just above the base of the 5th metatarsal.

NOTES:

BODY PART: Ankle

POSITION/PROJECTION: Anteroposterior

ANATOMY: An anteroposterior projection of the ankle joint, the distal tibia and fibula, and the proximal aspect of the talus.

PATIENT/PART POSITION: Dorsiflex the foot enough to place the long axis of the foot in the vertical position (plantar surface is perpendicular to the image receptor). Invert the foot approximately 5 to 15 degrees.

CENTRAL RAY LOCATION/ANGLE: The central ray is directed perpendicular to the ankle joint midway between the two malleoli.

NOTES:

BODY PART: Ankle

POSITION/PROJECTION: Medial Oblique

ANATOMY: The distal ends of the tibia and fibula, especially the lateral malleolus and ankle mortise.

PATIENT/PART POSITION: Have the patient dorsiflex the foot and rotate it internally (medially) 20 to 25 degrees to insure proper rotation of the ankle joint.

CENTRAL RAY LOCATION/ANGLE: The central ray is directed perpendicular to the ankle joint midway between the two malleoli.

NOTES:

BODY PART: Ankle

POSITION/PROJECTION: Lateral

ANATOMY: A lateral projection of the distal tibia and fibula, the ankle joint, and the talus. This view should include the base of the fifth metatarsal.

PATIENT/PART POSITION: Have the patient roll up towards the affected side and dorsiflex the foot. Both the leg and foot should be in the lateral position.

CENTRAL RAY LOCATION/ANGLE: The central ray is directed perpendicular to the mid-ankle joint.

NOTES:

BODY PART: Calcaneus

POSITION/PROJECTION: Lateral

ANATOMY: A lateral projection of the calcaneus.

PATIENT/PART POSITION: Have the patient roll up onto the affected side, placing the foot and ankle into the lateral position. Have the patient dorsiflex the foot. Place the center of the image receptor approximately 1 to 1½ inches below the medial malleolus.

CENTRAL RAY LOCATION/ANGLE: The central ray is directed perpendicular to the image receptor.

NOTES:

BODY PART: Calcaneus

POSITION/PROJECTION: Semiaxial

ANATOMY: An plantodorsal projection of the calcaneus from the tuberosity to the sustentaculum tali and trochlear process.

PATIENT/PART POSITION: Have the patient extend the leg and dorsiflex the foot so that its plantar surface is perpendicular to the image receptor. Place the far edge of the image receptor at the level of the heel.

CENTRAL RAY LOCATION/ANGLE: The central ray is directed 40 degrees cephalic to enter at the base of the 5th metatarsal.

NOTES:

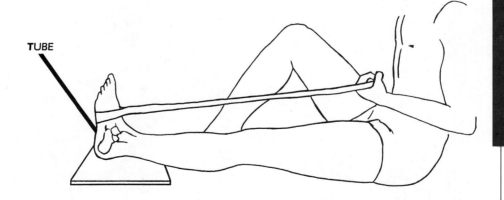

TUBE

Semiaxial **P**rojection of **C**alcaneus

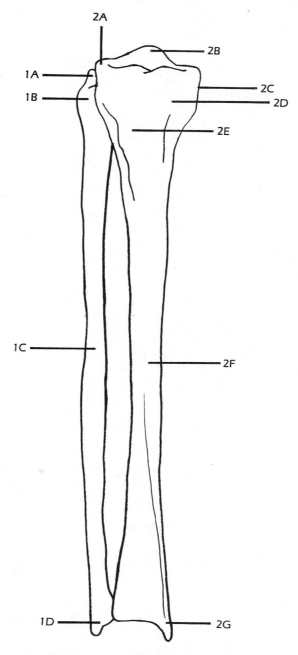

Anterior **A**spect of **F**ibula and **T**ibia

1. Fibula
   A. Styloid Process
   B. Head
   C. Shaft
   D. Lateral **M**alleolus

2. Tibia
   A. Lateral **C**ondyle
   B. Spines (**E**minence)
   C. Medial **C**ondyle
   D. Head
   E. Tibial **T**uberosity
   F. Shaft
   G. Medial **M**alleolus

BODY PART: Tibia and Fibula

POSITION/PROJECTION: Anteroposterior

ANATOMY: An anteroposterior projection of the tibia and fibula, including both the knee and the ankle joints.

PATIENT/PART POSITION: Place the patient's leg in the anteroposterior position with the toes pointing toward the ceiling; invert the foot slightly, but do not rotate the leg. The femoral condyles will be in a plane parallel to the floor.

CENTRAL RAY LOCATION/ANGLE: The central ray is directed perpendicular to the mid-shaft area.

NOTES:

BODY PART: Tibia and Fibula

POSITION/PROJECTION: Lateral

ANATOMY: A lateral projection of the tibia, fibula, and both the ankle and the knee joints.

PATIENT/PART POSITION: Rotate the patient toward the affected side until the leg is in a true lateral position.

CENTRAL RAY LOCATION/ANGLE: The central ray is directed perpendicular to the mid-shaft area.

NOTES:

BODY PART: Knee

POSITION/PROJECTION: Anteroposterior

ANATOMY: An anteroposterior projection of the bones and soft tissues of the knee, including the distal femur and patella, proximal tibia and fibula, and the interspace between the tibial plateau and the femoral condyles.

PATIENT/PART POSITION: Extend the knee fully. Adjust the leg to a true anteroposterior position; the patella will lie slightly to the medial side. Center the image receptor about ½ inch below the patellar apex.

CENTRAL RAY LOCATION/ANGLE: The central ray is angled 5 to 7 degrees cephalic when radiographing the joint space. It is perpendicular when performing radiography of the distal femur and proximal tibia and fibula. In either case, the central ray is directed to the midpoint of the image receptor.

NOTES:

BODY PART: Knee—Special Examinations (Intercondyloid Fossa)

POSITION/PROJECTION: Posteroanterior Axial—Camp-Coventry Method

ANATOMY: A superior-inferior projection of the intercondyloid fossa in a more "open" image.

PATIENT/PART POSITION: The patient is prone on the table. The knee is flexed 40 degrees, and the foot is rested on a suitable support.

CENTRAL RAY LOCATION/ANGLE: The central ray is directed 40 degrees caudal so that it is perpendicular to the long axis of the tibia and fibula and enters the popliteal depression.

NOTES:

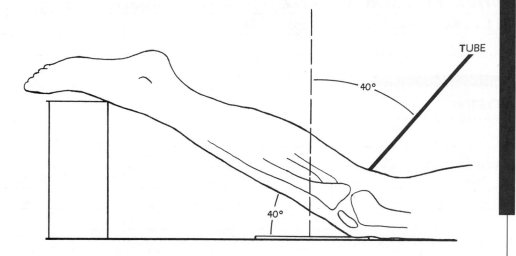

TUBE

40°

40°

Intercondyloid Fossa
PA Axial **P**osition

BODY PART: Knee—Special Examinations (Intercondyloid Fossa)

POSITION/PROJECTION: Anteroposterior Axial—Beclere Method

ANATOMY: A profile image of the intercondyloid fossa, the tibial spine, and the knee joint.

PATIENT/PART POSITION: The patient is supine on the table with affected knee flexed to place the long axis of the femur at a 60-degree angle to the long axis of the tibia. The knee is then supported and the image receptor placed under the knee.

CENTRAL RAY LOCATION/ANGLE: The central ray is directed perpendicular to the long axis of the tibia and centered to the knee joint.

NOTES:

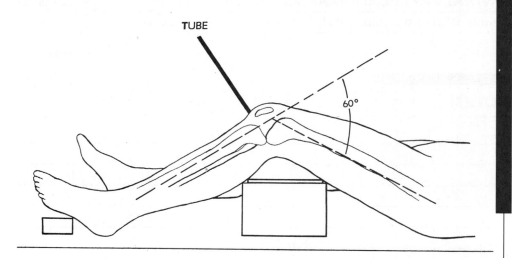

TUBE

60°

Intercondyloid **F**ossa
AP **A**xial **P**osition

BODY PART: Knee—Special Examinations (Intercondyloid Fossa)

POSITION/PROJECTION: Posteroanterior Axial—Holmblad Method

ANATOMY: The intercondyloid fossa of the femur and the tibial spine in profile.

PATIENT/PART POSITION: The patient is kneeling on the table so that the long axis of the femur forms an angle of 70 degrees (from the horizontal) with the plane of the table.

CENTRAL RAY LOCATION/ANGLE: The central ray is directed perpendicular to the midpoint of the film, which is centered to the patellar apex.

NOTES:

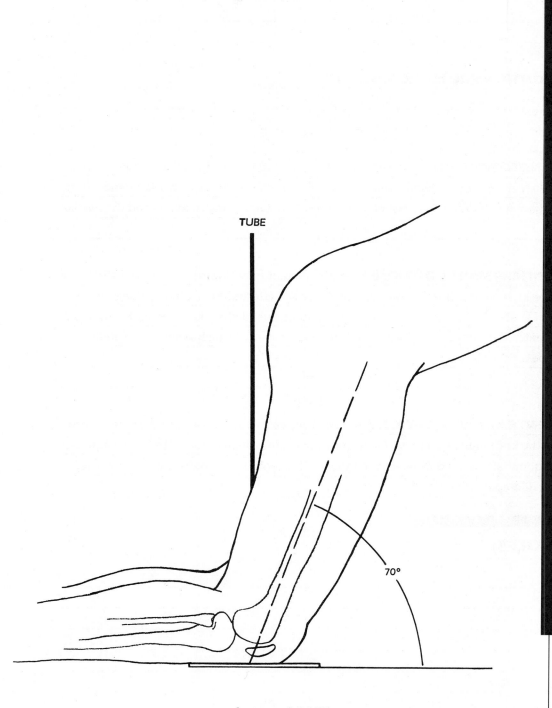

TUBE

70°

Intercondyloid Fossa
PA Axial Position

BODY PART: Knee

POSITION/PROJECTION: Lateral

ANATOMY: A lateral projection of the distal femur, the patella, the joint space between the tibial plateau and the femoral condyles, the proximal tibia and fibula, adjacent soft tissue, and the interspace between the femoral condyles and the patella.

PATIENT/PART POSITION: Have the patient turn toward the affected side until the knee is in a true lateral position. Flex the affected knee 20 to 30 degrees. The ankle should be supported to keep the long axis of the tibia parallel to the table. Center the image receptor to the knee joint, about ½ inch below the patellar apex.

CENTRAL RAY LOCATION/ANGLE: The central ray is directed 5 degrees cephalic to the knee joint. This prevents the joint space from being obscured by the magnified shadow of the medial femoral condyle. The central ray enters 1 cm below the medial epicondyle.

NOTES:

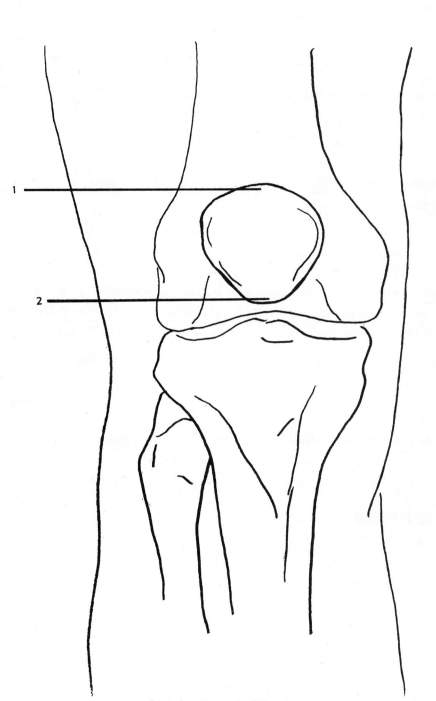

Anterior **A**spect of **P**atella

1. Base   **2. A**pex

BODY PART: Knee (Patella)

POSITION/PROJECTION: Tangential—Settegast Method

ANATOMY: Vertical fractures of the patella and the articulating surfaces of the femoro-patellar articulations.

PATIENT/PART POSITION: The patient is placed prone on the table. The affected knee is slowly flexed until the patella is perpendicular to the film. **NOT TO BE USED WITH SUSPECTED HORIZONTAL FRACTURES OF THE PATELLA.**

CENTRAL RAY LOCATION/ANGLE: The central ray is directed perpendicular to the joint space between the patella and the femoral condyles. The degree of angulation of the tube depends on the degree of flexion of the knee.

NOTES:

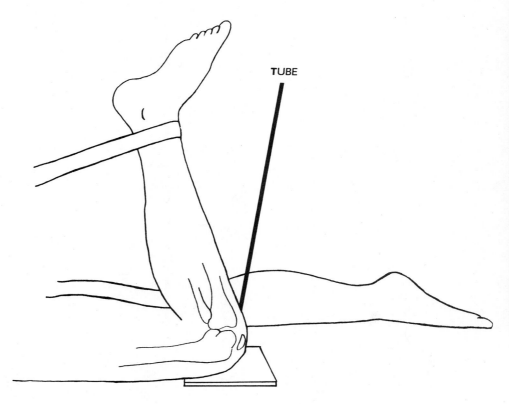

Patella
Tangential **P**osition

TUBE

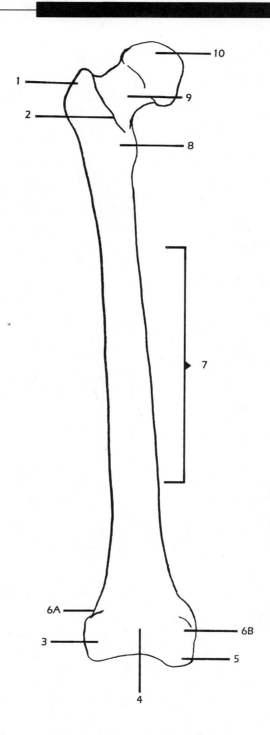

Anterior Aspect of Femur

1. Greater Trochanter
2. Intertrochanteric Crest
3. Lateral Condyle
4. Articular Surface for the Patella
5. Medial Condyle
6. Epicondyle
   A. Lateral
   B. Medial
7. Shaft
8. Lesser Trochanter
9. Neck
10. Head

BODY PART: Femur

POSITION/PROJECTION: Anteroposterior

ANATOMY: A anteroposterior view of the femur including the hip and/or knee joint.

PATIENT/PART POSITION: In cases of suspected fracture(s), the leg should be radiographed in position and the film checked by a physician. **DO NOT CHANGE THE POSITION OF THE LEG UNTIL APPROVED BY A PHYSICIAN.** Invert the feet 15 degrees to overcome anteversion of the femoral neck. Place the top of the image receptor 2 inches above the greater trochanter for the proximal femur. For the distal femur, place the bottom of the image receptor 2 inches below the knee joint.

CENTRAL RAY LOCATION/ANGLE: Direct the central ray to the midpoint of the image receptor.

NOTES:

BODY PART: Femur

POSITION/PROJECTION: Lateral—Lower Femur

ANATOMY: A lateral projection of the distal femur and the knee joint.

PATIENT/PART POSITION: Have the patient roll up on the affected side. Draw the upper leg forward; flex the affected knee; place the leg so that the patella is perpendicular to the table. Adjust the image receptor in the Bucky tray so that the lower border is 2 inches below the knee joint.

CENTRAL RAY LOCATION/ANGLE: The central ray is directed to the midpoint of the image receptor.

NOTES:

BODY PART: Femur

POSITION/PROJECTION: Upper Femur Lateral—Frog Leg

ANATOMY: An axial projection of the femoral head, neck, and trochanteric area.

PATIENT/PART POSITION: Have the patient flex the knee, fully abducting the thigh so that it is contact with the table. This will require that the patient be slightly obliqued posteriorly on to the affected side. The femoral neck is centered to the midline of the table.

CENTRAL RAY LOCATION/ANGLE: The central ray is directed perpendicular to the femoral neck and to the midpoint of the image receptor.

NOTES:

BODY PART: Hip

POSITION/PROJECTION: Translateral—Danielus-Miller Method

ANATOMY: A translateral projection of the proximal femur, including the head, neck, and trochanters of the femur and the acetabulum of the pelvis.

PATIENT/PART POSITION: Using folded sheets or sponges, elevate the affected hip so that the most prominent point of the greater trochanter is centered to the image receptor. A stationary grid cassette is used for this position. It is placed vertically next to the patient's affected side, so that the upper vertical border of the cassette is pressed into the soft tissue above the iliac crest. Localize the long axis of the femoral neck by visualizing a line between the anterior superior iliac spine and the upper border of the symphysis pubis. Note the center of this line. Localize a point 1 inch medial to the most prominent lateral point of the greater trochanter. The intersecting line between the line and the point will parallel the long axis of the femoral neck. Flex the unaffected leg and hip to avoid superimposition with the central ray and hip joint being radiographed. A 15-degree internal rotation of the affected leg will provide a profile of the femoral neck. **THIS ROTATION SHOULD BE DONE ONLY AFTER CAREFUL ASSESSMENT OF THE PATIENT'S CONDITION.**

CENTRAL RAY LOCATION/ANGLE: The tube is placed in a horizontal position. The central ray is perpendicular to the long axis of the femoral neck and directed to the midpoint of the image receptor.

NOTES:

Check that the central ray is perpendicular to the grid cassette and that the grid cassette is perpendicular to the horizontal plane when performing a cross-table lateral.

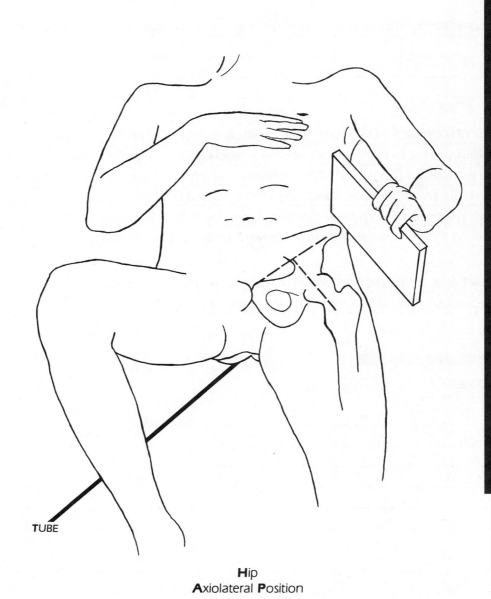

TUBE

Hip
Axiolateral **P**osition

BODY PART: Hip

POSITION/PROJECTION: Anteroposterior Axial—Modified Cleaves Method

ANATOMY: An axial projection of the femoral head, neck, and trochanteric area.

PATIENT/PART POSITION: This position should NEVER be attempted on a trauma patient. In cases where a fracture is suspected or a history of fracture is noted, the translateral (Danielus-Miller method) is substituted for the Cleaves method. Have the patient flex the knee, fully abducting the thigh so that it is in contact with the table. This requires that the patient be slightly obliqued onto the affected side. The femoral neck is centered to the midline of the table.

CENTRAL RAY LOCATION/ANGLE: The central ray is directed perpendicular to the femoral neck and to the midpoint of the image receptor.

NOTES:

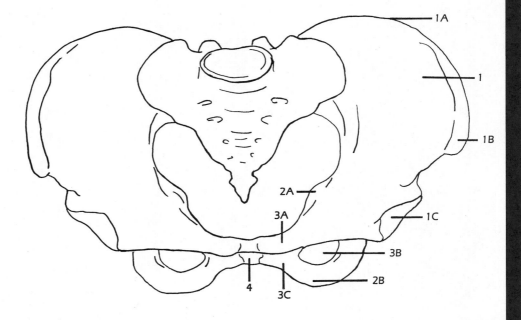

Anterior Aspect of Pelvis

1. Ilium
  A. Crest
  B. Anterior Superior Iliac Spine
  C. Anterior Inferior Iliac Spine
2. Ischium
  A. Ischial Spine
  B. Ischial Tuberosity

3. Pubis
  A. Superior Ramus
  B. Obturator Foramen
  C. Inferior Ramus
4. Symphysis Pubis

BODY PART: Pelvis

POSITION/PROJECTION: Anteroposterior

ANATOMY: An anteroposterior projection of the pelvic girdle and the head, neck, trochanter, and upper third or fourth of the femoral shaft.

PATIENT/PART POSITION: Center the midsagittal plane of the entire body to the midline of the table. Invert the feet 15 degrees to overcome the anteversion of the femoral necks. **(Use caution with suspected hip fractures).** With the image receptor in the Bucky tray, adjust it so that its upper border is 1 to 1½ inches above the top of the iliac crest.

CENTRAL RAY LOCATION/ANGLE: The central ray is directed to the midpoint of the image receptor.

NOTES:

PART
3

Thorax

Chest 103

Ribs 117

Sternum 121

Sternoclavicular Joints 123

THORAX

GENERAL TECHNICAL TIPS: DID YOU REMEMBER TO?

- ◼ properly identify the patient?

- ◼ ask a female patient if she may be pregnant?

- ◼ get an accurate history from the patient?

- ◼ determine whether the exam is being performed as the result of trauma or to detect pathology?

- ◼ remove all opaque objects and clothing from the area of interest?

- ◼ properly shield the patient?

- ◼ check breathing instructions with the patient?

- ◼ use the proper markers on the film (i.e., erect, semierect, supine, right, left, and other appropriate markers)?

- ◼ collimate to the part?

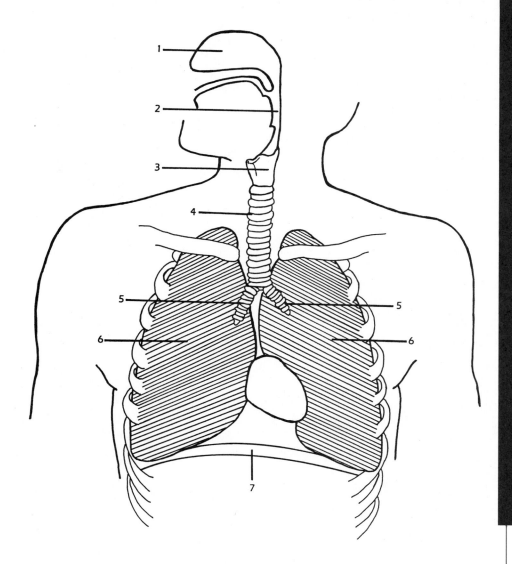

Anterior **A**spect of **R**espiratory **S**ystem

1. **N**asal **C**avity
2. **P**harynx
3. **L**arynx
4. **T**rachea

5. **P**rimary **B**ronchi
6. **L**ungs
7. **D**iaphragm

BODY PART: Chest

POSITION/PROJECTION: Posteroanterior

ANATOMY: A posteroanterior projection of the thoracic viscera including an air-filled trachea, lungs, diaphragmatic domes, heart, and aortic knob.

PATIENT/PART POSITION: Center the midsagittal plane of the body to the midline of the image receptor or upright Bucky. Place the top of the image receptor 1½ inches above the shoulders. Place the hands on the hips low enough so they will not be superimposed on the costophrenic angles and, with the palms rotated outward, rotate the shoulders and elbows toward the image receptor.

CENTRAL RAY LOCATION/ANGLE: The central ray is directed to the midsagittal plane at the level of the 6th thoracic vertebra.

NOTES:

BODY PART: Chest

POSITION/PROJECTION: Left Lateral

ANATOMY: A left lateral projection of the heart, aorta, and left-sided pulmonary lesions. It also demonstrates interlobar fissures.

PATIENT/PART POSITION: Place the thorax with the left side against the image receptor so that the midaxillary line is 2 inches posterior to its midline. Direct the patient to extend the arms upward, flexing the elbows and, resting the forearms on the head, grasp each elbow with the opposite hand.

CENTRAL RAY LOCATION/ANGLE: The central ray is directed horizontally and centered at the level of the 6th thoracic vertebra.

NOTES:

BODY PART: Chest—Special Examinations

POSITION/PROJECTION: Right Lateral

ANATOMY: Right-sided pulmonary lesions and right interlobar fissures.

PATIENT/PART POSITION: Place the thorax with the right side against the image receptor so that the midaxillary line is 2 inches posterior to its midline. Direct the patient to extend the arms upward, flexing the elbows and, resting the forearms on the head, grasp each elbow with the opposite hand.

CENTRAL RAY LOCATION/ANGLE: The central ray is directed horizontally and centered at the level of the 6th thoracic vertebra.

NOTES:

BODY PART: Chest—Special Examinations

POSITION/PROJECTION: Right Anterior Oblique

ANATOMY: The heart and thoracic aorta, free from superimposition of the spine. Air-filled trachea and its bifurcation, the right lung field, and a foreshortened view of the left lung.

PATIENT/PART POSITION: Place the anterior surface of the patient's right shoulder against the upright Bucky, keeping the image receptor 1½ inches above the shoulder. Rotate the left side away from the upright Bucky until it forms an angle of 45 degrees. Place the patient's left hand on top of the upright Bucky and place the right hand, palm out, on the right hip. Center the thoracic cavity to the upright Bucky device.

CENTRAL RAY LOCATION/ANGLE: The central ray is directed to the center of the thoracic cavity at the level of the 6th thoracic vertebra.

NOTES:

BODY PART: Chest—Special Examinations

POSITION/PROJECTION: Left Anterior Oblique

ANATOMY: The greatest portion of the left lung field, projected free of superimposition of the spine, as well as the trachea and entire left branch of bronchial tree. Also demonstrates a foreshortened view of the right lung and the right retrocardial space.

PATIENT/PART POSITION: Place the anterior surface of the patient's left shoulder against the upright Bucky, keeping the image receptor 1½ inches above the shoulder. Rotate the right side away from the upright Bucky until it forms an angle of 45 degrees.* Place the patient's right hand on top of the upright Bucky and place the left hand, palm out, on the left hip. Center the thoracic cavity to the upright Bucky device.

CENTRAL RAY LOCATION/ANGLE: The central ray is directed to the midsagittal plane at the level of the 6th thoracic vertebra.

NOTES:

*Use 45 degrees for routine exams, 55 to 60 degrees may be used for studies of the heart and great vessels.

_____

BODY PART: Chest—Special Examinations

_____

_____

_____

POSITION/PROJECTION: Right Posterior Oblique

_____

_____

_____

ANATOMY: The greatest portion of the left lung field, projected free of super-imposition of the spine, as well as trachea and entire right branch of bronchial tree. Also demonstrates a foreshortened view of the right lung and the left retrocardial space.

PATIENT/PART POSITION: Place patient's right scapula against the upright Bucky, keeping the image receptor 1½ inches above the shoulder. Rotate the left side away from upright Bucky until it forms an angle of 45 degrees. Elevate the patient's right arm and place the hand behind the head. Place the patient's left hand, palm out, on the left hip. Center the thoracic cavity to the upright Bucky.

CENTRAL RAY LOCATION/ANGLE: The central ray is directed to the midsagittal plane at the level of the 6th thoracic vertebra.

_____

NOTES:
_____

_____

_____

_____

_____

_____

_____

_____

_____

_____

_____

BODY PART: Chest—Special Examinations

POSITION/PROJECTION: Left Posterior Oblique

ANATOMY: The heart and thoracic aorta free from superimposition of the spine. Air-filled trachea and its bifurcation, the greatest portion of the right lung field, and the foreshortened view of the left lung.

PATIENT/PART POSITION: Place the posterior surface of the patient's left shoulder against the upright Bucky, keeping the image receptor 1½ inches above the shoulder. Rotate the right side away from the upright Bucky until it forms an angle of 45 degrees. Raise the patient's right arm, flexing the elbow, and place the patient's right hand behind the head. Place the left hand, palm out, on the left hip. Center the thoracic cavity to the upright Bucky device.

CENTRAL RAY LOCATION/ANGLE: The central ray is directed to the midsagittal plane at the level of the 6th thoracic vertebra.

NOTES:

BODY PART: Chest—Special Examinations

POSITION/PROJECTION: Anteroposterior Lordotic

ANATOMY: An AP axial projection of the lungs which is used to demonstrate the apices (smaller-size film) and such conditions as interlobar effusions (full-size film).

PATIENT/PART POSITION: Place the patient in the AP position, at a distance of approximately 1 foot in front of the upright grid device. Lean the patient back, centering the midsagittal plane to the midline of the vertical Bucky with the shoulders, neck, and back of the head against the upright Bucky. Adjust the upright Bucky so that the upper margin of the image receptor will be about 3 inches above the shoulders. Reposition the patient and rest both hands on the hips, palms out, and roll the shoulders forward, keeping the upper portion of the posterior thorax resting against the upright Bucky.

CENTRAL RAY LOCATION/ANGLE: The central ray is directed horizontally to the midpoint of the image receptor.

NOTES:

BODY PART: Chest—Special Examinations

POSITION/PROJECTION: Anteroposterior Sitting

ANATOMY: An AP projection of the thoracic viscera in the semierect position. It is employed when a patient is too ill or physically unable to stand but when air and fluid levels must be detected.

PATIENT/PART POSITION: Place the patient in the AP position erect. Adjust the image receptor so that its upper end rests 1½ to 2½ inches above the shoulders and center the midsagittal plane to the center of the image receptor.

CENTRAL RAY LOCATION/ANGLE: The central ray is directed perpendicularly to the image receptor to enter the middle of the patient's sternum.

NOTES:

The x-ray beam **MUST** be parallel to the floor in order to demonstrate air/fluid levels.

BODY PART: Chest—Special Examinations

POSITION/PROJECTION: Supine

ANATOMY: Anteroposterior projection of the thoracic viscera in the supine position. It is employed when a patient is too ill or physically unable to sit or stand. It will not demonstrate air or fluid levels but may be used to localize pulmonary lesions; tubes, lines, and catheters entering the chest cavity; and endotracheal tubes.

PATIENT/PART POSITION: With the patient supine, place the image receptor in the Bucky device or directly under the patient (as in stretcher or portable exams). Adjust the image receptor so that the upper border is 1½ to 2½ inches above the shoulders, centered to the midsagittal plane.

CENTRAL RAY LOCATION/ANGLE: The central ray is directed perpendicular to the image receptor, entering at the middle of the patient's sternum.

NOTES:

BODY PART: Chest—Special Examinations

POSITION/PROJECTION: Lateral Decubitus

ANATOMY: Left and right lateral decubitus positions (AP or PA projections) demonstrate small pleural effusions and/or air/fluid levels in the pleural space.

PATIENT/PART POSITION: The patient lies on the left side (for left lateral decubitus) or right side (for right lateral decubitus). Both arms are raised above the head with anterior or posterior surface of the patient's thorax in contact with an upright grid device or image receptor. Center the thorax to the image receptor and adjust the patient to place the image receptor 2 to 3 inches above the patient's shoulders.

CENTRAL RAY LOCATION/ANGLE: The central ray is directed horizontally to the midpoint of the image receptor.

NOTES:

The x-ray beam **MUST** be parallel to the floor in order to demonstrate air/fluid levels.

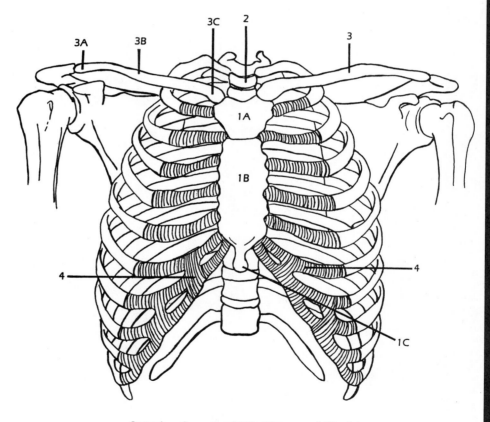

Anterior **A**spect of **R**ib **C**age and **C**lavicle

1. Sternum
   A. **M**anubrium
   B. **B**ody
   C. **X**iphoid **P**rocess
2. **T**horacic **V**ertebrae

3. **C**lavicle
   A. **A**cromial or **L**ateral **E**nd
   B. **S**haft
   C. **S**ternal or **M**edial **E**nd
4. **C**ostal **C**artilage

BODY PART: Ribs

POSITION/PROJECTION: Anteroposterior—Ribs above the Diaphragm

ANATOMY: An AP projection of the ribs (posterior) closest to the film and above the diaphragm.

PATIENT/PART POSITION: The midsagittal plane is centered to the midline of the film for a bilateral projection of the ribs. For a unilateral projection, the side of interest is centered midway between the axillary border and the midsagittal plane. The image receptor is positioned so that the upper edge is 1½ inches above the top of the shoulder.

CENTRAL RAY LOCATION/ANGLE: The central ray enters at the level of the 6th thoracic vertebra.

NOTES:

BODY PART: Ribs

POSITION/PROJECTION: Anteroposterior—Ribs below the Diaphragm

ANATOMY: An AP projection of the ribs closest to the film (posterior) and below the diaphragm.

PATIENT/PART POSITION: For bilateral ribs, center the midsagittal plane to the midline of the image receptor. For unilateral ribs, center midway between the midsagittal plane and the axillary border of the side in question. In either situation, the image receptor is centered to the 12th thoracic vertebra.

CENTRAL RAY LOCATION/ANGLE: The central ray enters at the level of the 12th thoracic vertebra.

NOTES:

BODY PART: Ribs

POSITION/PROJECTION: Right and Left Posterior Obliques—Ribs above the Diaphragm

ANATOMY: The axillary portion of the ribs above the diaphragm, free of superimposition from the other portions of the ribs.

PATIENT/PART POSITION: The patient is rotated 45 degrees from the supine or erect AP position towards the affected side and is centered to a plane midway between the midsagittal plane and the axillary border of the patient. The image receptor is placed so that the upper edge is 1½ inches above the top of the shoulder.

CENTRAL RAY LOCATION/ANGLE: The central ray enters at the level of the 6th thoracic vertebra.

NOTES:

The LAO and RAO positions may also be used for examinations of the ribs. The LAO and RPO demonstrate the same anatomy: the RAO and LPO demonstrate the same anatomy.

BODY PART: Ribs

POSITION/PROJECTION: Right and Left Posterior Obliques—Ribs below the Diaphragm

ANATOMY: An AP projection of the axillary portion of the ribs below the diaphragm so that they are free of superimposition from the other portions of the ribs.

PATIENT/PART POSITION: The patient is positioned the same as the AP oblique projection above the diaphragms. The image receptor is placed so that it is centered at the level of the 12th thoracic vertebra.

CENTRAL RAY LOCATION/ANGLE: The central ray enters at the level of the 12th thoracic vertebra and is centered to the image receptor.

NOTES:

The LAO and RAO positions may also be used for examinations of the ribs. The LAO and RPO demonstrate the same anatomy: the RAO and LPO demonstrate the same anatomy.

BODY PART: Sternum

POSITION/PROJECTION: Right Anterior Oblique

ANATOMY: An oblique PA projection of the sternum which is free of superimposition from the spine.

PATIENT/PART POSITION: The patient is placed either prone on the table or facing the upright Bucky. Rotate the patient to a 15- to 20-degree right anterior oblique position so that the sternum is centered to the midline of the table.

CENTRAL RAY LOCATION/ANGLE: The central ray is directed at right angles to a point midway between the manubrial notch and the xiphoid tip.

NOTES:

A quiet breathing technique may be utilized to blur the lung shadows.

BODY PART: Sternum

POSITION/PROJECTION: Left Lateral

ANATOMY: A lateral projection of the sternum, the medial ends of the clavicles, and the sternoclavicular joints superimposed.

PATIENT/PART POSITION: Have the patient stand erect against the upright Bucky in a left lateral position. Place the top of the image receptor 1½ inches above the manubrial notch. Rotate the patient's shoulders posteriorly and place the hands behind the back, this will remove superimposition of the shoulders and sternum.

CENTRAL RAY LOCATION/ANGLE: The central ray is directed at right angles to the midpoint of the sternum.

NOTES:

BODY PART: Sternoclavicular Joints

POSITION/PROJECTION: Posteroanterior

ANATOMY: A PA projection of the sternoclavicular joints and the medial one-third of the clavicles.

PATIENT/PART POSITION: Place the patient prone on the table or erect facing an upright Bucky. Center the midsagittal plane to the midline of the table or the upright Bucky. Center the image receptor to the level of the manubrial notch.

CENTRAL RAY LOCATION/ANGLE: The central ray is directed perpendicular to the center of the image receptor.

NOTES:

BODY PART: Sternoclavicular Joints

POSITION/PROJECTION: Right and Left Anterior Obliques

ANATOMY: A slight oblique projection of the sternoclavicular joint closest to the image receptor.

PATIENT/PART POSITION: The patient is prone or erect facing an upright Bucky, with the affected joint adjacent to the image receptor. Slightly oblique the patient, away from the affected side so that the vertebral shadow is not in alignment with the affected sternoclavicular joint and the joint is centered to the image receptor. (This will result in an angle of 15 degrees with the midsagittal plane of the body). The image receptor is centered to the sternoclavicular joint.

CENTRAL RAY LOCATION/ANGLE: The central ray enters perpendicularly to the midpoint of the image receptor, exiting from the affected sternoclavicular joint.

NOTES:

PART
4

Abdomen

Abdomen 127

ABDOMEN

GENERAL TECHNICAL TIPS:
DID YOU
REMEMBER TO?

- properly identify the patient?

- ask a female patient if she may be pregnant?

- use the ten-day rule in cases of suspected pregnancy?

- request information from the patient to determine reason(s) for doing the exam?

- remove any opaque objects from the field of interest?

- use the table pad for the patient's comfort?

- respect the patient's modesty by providing linen to properly cover the patient?

- explain the breathing instructions to the patient?

- use the proper markers on the film (erect, supine, decubitus, right, left, and others as needed)?

- collimate to the part (if possible)?

- properly shield the patient (if possible)?

BODY PART: Abdomen

POSITION/PROJECTION: Anteroposterior—Supine

ANATOMY: An anteroposterior projection of the abdomen showing the size and shape of the liver, spleen, and kidneys and any intraabdominal calcifications or tumor masses.

PATIENT/PART POSITION: The patient is placed in a supine position with the midsagittal plane of the body centered to the midline of the table. The image receptor is centered to level of the iliac crest.

CENTRAL RAY LOCATION/ANGLE: The central ray is directed to the midpoint of the image receptor.

NOTES:

BODY PART: Abdomen

POSITION/PROJECTION: Anteroposterior—Erect

ANATOMY: An anteroposterior projection of the abdomen showing the size and shape of the liver, spleen, and kidneys and any intraabdominal calcifications or tumor masses. It also demonstrates the presence of air/fluid levels within the small or large intestines.

PATIENT/PART POSITION: The patient is placed in the erect anteroposterior position with the midsagittal plane of the body centered to the midline of the vertical grid device. Center the image receptor 2 to 3 inches above the iliac crest in order to include hemidiaphragms.

CENTRAL RAY LOCATION/ANGLE: The central ray is directed to the midpoint of the image receptor. If the patient is unable to stand, the left lateral decubitus position is used in lieu of this position.

NOTES:

In order to demonstrate air/fluid levels, the central ray **MUST** be parallel to the floor.

BODY PART: Abdomen

POSITION/PROJECTION: Left Lateral Decubitus

ANATOMY: Intraperitoneal gas and air/fluid levels within the abdomen. Free air will rise under the right hemidiaphragm where it will not be obscured by the gastric gas bubble.

PATIENT/PART POSITION: Place the patient on a stretcher lying on the left side. Then position the stretcher against the vertical grid device and lock it. Center the image receptor to the midsagittal plane 2 inches above the level of the iliac crests.

CENTRAL RAY LOCATION/ANGLE: The central ray is directed perpendicular to the center of the image receptor.

NOTES:

In order to demonstrate air/fluid levels, the central ray **MUST** be parallel to the floor.

BODY PART: Abdomen

POSITION/PROJECTION: Cross-Table Lateral—Dorsal Decubitus

ANATOMY: The antevertebral space occupied by the abdominal aorta, as well as any intraabdominal calcifications, tumor masses, and umbilical hernias.

PATIENT/PART POSITION: With the patient supine on a stretcher, place the stretcher against the vertical grid device and lock it. Move the patient toward the upright Bucky till the left side of the patient is in contact with the Bucky. Raise both the patient's arms above the head. The image receptor is centered at the level of the iliac crests midway between the anterior and posterior surfaces of the body.

CENTRAL RAY LOCATION/ANGLE: The central ray is directed horizontally to the midpoint of the image receptor. This projection can also be performed on the x-ray table, but a grid must be used with the image receptor.

NOTES:

PART
5

Abdomen with Contrast Media

Urinary System 134

Biliary System 144

Gastrointestinal System 152

Barium Enema 166

ABDOMEN WITH CONTRAST MEDIA

GENERAL TECHNICAL TIPS:
DID YOU
REMEMBER TO?

■ properly identify the patient?

■ ask a female patient if she may be pregnant?

■ use the ten-day rule in cases of suspected pregnancy?

■ request information from the patient to determine reason(s) for performing the exam?

■ use a table pad for the patient's comfort?

■ repect the patient's modesty by providing linen to properly cover the patient?

■ check the contrast media and the patient's condition to avoid any contraindicated situation?

■ properly prepare the contrast media used?

■ be prepared for allergic and/or other reactions during administration of the contrast media?

■ explain the exam to the patient?

■ record the time of administration of the contrast media and utilize time markers on each radiograph?

■ collimate to the part (if possible)?

■ properly shield the patient (if possible)?

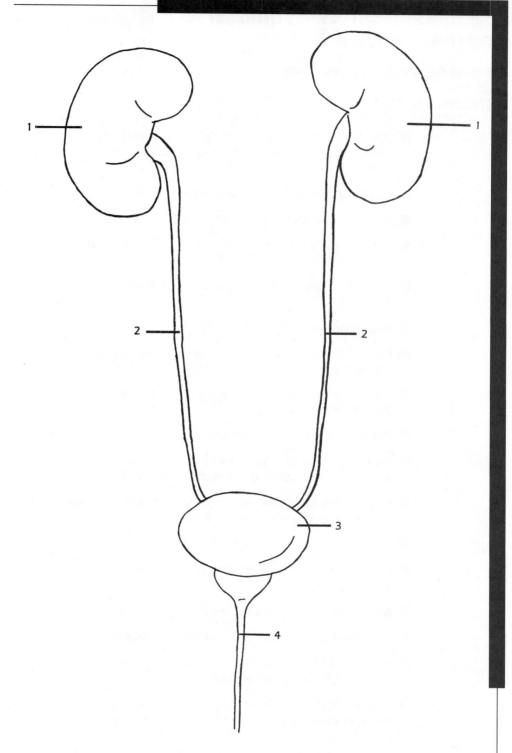

Anterior **A**spect of **U**rinary **S**ystem

1. Kidney   **2. U**reter   **3. U**rinary **B**ladder   **4. U**rethra

URINARY SYSTEM

GENERAL TECHNICAL TIPS:
DID YOU
REMEMBER TO?

■ check with the patient for allergies and medications taken and elicit a history describing the reason for the exam?

■ check that the consent form has been signed?

■ check for urinary catheter and/or IV?

■ have the patient empty his or her bladder before the exam begins?

■ check the emergency cart's location and the status of its supplies?

■ have a emesis basin ready?

■ have all the necessary supplies on hand for the administration of the contrast media?

■ use sterile technique for drawing up and administering the contrast media?

■ introduce the doctor to the patient?

■ record the time of administration of the contrast media and utilize time markers on each radiograph?

■ be prepared for a contrast-media reaction and be aware of the contraindications of the media?

■ use the proper markers on each film?

■ turn the patient's head to the side if nausea and vomiting occur?

■ check your exposure factors, especially KVP?

■ have compression apparatus available if needed?

■ communicate clearly with the doctor(s) performing and assisting with the examination?

■ have enough protective aprons available for any personnel who need to remain in the room during the exam?

BODY PART: Urinary System—Excretory Urography

POSITION/PROJECTION: Anteroposterior—Scout

ANATOMY: An anteroposterior projection of the kidneys, ureters, urinary bladder, and surrounding organs and structures.

PATIENT/PART POSITION: The patient is supine with the midsagittal plane centered to the midline of the table. The image receptor is centered to the level of the iliac crests, its bottom edge at the level of the symphysis pubis.

CENTRAL RAY LOCATION/ANGLE: The central ray is directed perpendicular to the midpoint of the image receptor.

NOTES:

BODY PART: Urinary System—Excretory Urography

POSITION/PROJECTION: Anteroposterior—Postinjection of Contrast

ANATOMY: An anteroposterior projection of the kidneys, ureters, and bladder filled with contrast material.

PATIENT/PART POSITION: The patient is supine with the midsagittal plane centered to the midline of the table. The patient's arms are placed by his side. The image receptor is centered to the level of the iliac crests, its bottom edge at the level of the symphysis pubis.

CENTRAL RAY LOCATION/ANGLE: The central ray is directed perpendicular to the midpoint of the image receptor.

NOTES:

BODY PART: Urinary System—Excretory Urography

POSITION/PROJECTION: Anteroposterior—Cone Down of Kidneys

ANATOMY: An anteroposterior projection of the kidneys and proximal ureters filled with contrast material.

PATIENT/PART POSITION: The patient is supine with the midsagittal plane centered to the midline of the table. The position of the kidneys (usually from T12 to L2) should be checked on the full AP image prior to cone down.

CENTRAL RAY LOCATION/ANGLE: The central ray is directed perpendicular to the midpoint of the image receptor.

NOTES:

BODY PART: Urinary System—Excretory Urography

POSITION/PROJECTION: Right and Left Posterior Obliques

ANATOMY: The right posterior oblique (RPO) position demonstrates the left kidney in profile and the right kidney and ureter free of superimposition from the spine. The left posterior oblique (LPO) position demonstrates the right right kidney in profile and the left kidney and ureter free of superimposition.

PATIENT/PART POSITION: The patient is supine on the table and rotated 30 degrees toward the desired side. Center the spine to the midline of the table and position the image receptor at the level of the iliac crests.

CENTRAL RAY LOCATION/ANGLE: The central ray is directed perpendicular to the center of the image receptor.

NOTES:

BODY PART: Urinary System—Excretory Urography

POSITION/PROJECTION: Anteroposterior—Cone Down of the Bladder

ANATOMY: An anteroposterior projection of the bladder and distal ureters. This examination may be done pre void or post void.

PATIENT/PART POSITION: The patient is supine on the table with the midsagittal plane centered to the midline of the table and to a point midway between the anterior superior iliac spine and the symphysis pubis. The bottom of the image receptor is placed just above the greater trochanters.

CENTRAL RAY LOCATION/ANGLE: The central ray is directed perpendicular to the center of the image receptor.

NOTES:

BODY PART: Urinary System—Cystography

POSITION/PROJECTION: Anteroposterior

ANATOMY: The urinary bladder, the proximal urethra, and the distal third of the ureters filled with contrast material.

PATIENT/PART POSITION: The midsagittal plane is centered to the midline of the image receptor. Center the image receptor to a transverse plane 1½ inches above the symphysis pubis.

CENTRAL RAY LOCATION/ANGLE: The central ray is directed perpendicular to the center of the image receptor.

NOTES:

BODY PART: Urinary System—Cystography

POSITION/PROJECTION: Right and Left Posterior Oblique

ANATOMY: An anteroposterior oblique projection of the bladder, the proximal urethra, and a profile of the distal ureter closest to the film.

PATIENT/PART POSITION: The patient is rotated 40 to 60 degrees from the supine position towards either side. Center the patient to a sagittal plane 1 inch medial from the anterior superior iliac spine on the elevated side. The image receptor is centered to a point 1½ inches above the symphysis pubis.

CENTRAL RAY LOCATION/ANGLE: The central ray is directed perpendicular to the midpoint of the image receptor.

NOTES:

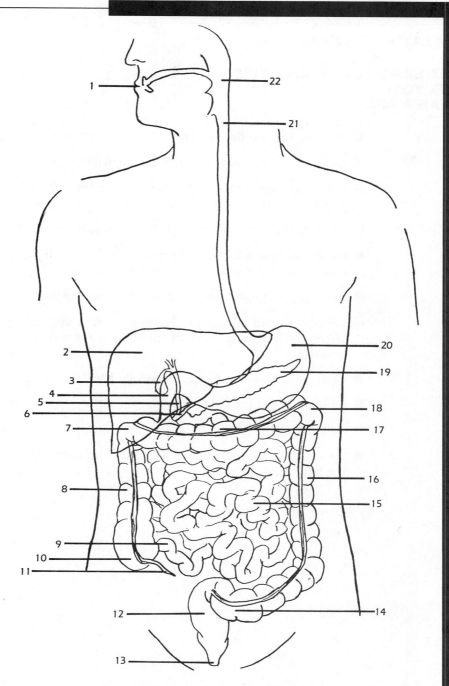

Anterior **A**spect of **D**igestive **S**ystem

1. **M**outh
2. **L**iver
3. **G**all **B**ladder
4. **D**uodenum
5. **C**ommon **B**ile **D**uct
6. **P**ancreatic **D**uct
7. **H**epatic **F**lexure

8. **A**scending **C**olon
9. **I**leum
10. **C**ecum
11. **V**ermiform **A**ppendix
12. **R**ectum
13. **A**nus
14. **S**igmoid **C**olon
15. **J**ejunum

16. **D**escending **C**olon
17. **T**ransverse **C**olon
18. **S**plenic **F**lexure
19. **P**ancreas
20. **S**tomach
21. **E**sophagus
22. **P**harynx

BILIARY SYSTEM

GENERAL TECHNICAL TIPS:
DID YOU
REMEMBER TO?

- ■ properly identify the patient?

- ■ ask a female patient if she may be pregnant?

- ■ check the patient's history i.e., does he or she still have a gall bladder?

- ■ check to see if the patient took the contrast media?

- ■ ask if the patient followed the prep and find out if there were any reactions to the contrast media?

- ■ use a pad to provide for the comfort of the patient?

- ■ perform a scout radiograph, keeping in mind that different bodily habitus affect the position of the gall bladder?

- ■ check your exposure factors, especially KVP?

- ■ properly shield the patient?

- ■ collimate to the part?

- ■ get the doctor's authorization **BEFORE** administering the fatty meal?

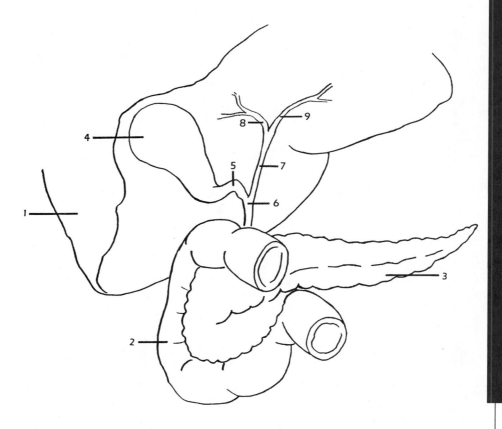

Anterior **A**spect of **B**iliary **S**ystem

1. Liver
2. Duodenum
3. Pancreas

4. Gall Bladder
5. Cystic Duct
6. Common Bile Duct

7. Common Hepatic Duct
8. Right Hepatic Duct
9. Left Hepatic Duct

BODY PART: Biliary System—Oral Cholecystography

POSITION/PROJECTION: Posteroanterior—Recumbent (Scout Film)

ANATOMY: To check for visualization and position of the gall bladder as well as general preparation of the abdomen.

PATIENT/PART POSITION: The patient is prone on the table with the midsagittal plane and iliac crests centered to the image receptor.

CENTRAL RAY LOCATION/ANGLE: The central ray is directed perpendicular to the center of the image receptor.

NOTES:

BODY PART: Biliary System—Oral Cholecystography

POSITION/PROJECTION: Posteroanterior—Recumbent

ANATOMY: Posteroanterior projection of the opacified gall bladder.

PATIENT/PART POSITION: The patient is prone on the table with the gall bladder area centered to the image receptor (determined from PA scout).

CENTRAL RAY LOCATION/ANGLE: The central ray is directed perpendicular to the midpoint of the image receptor.

NOTES:

BODY PART: Biliary System—Oral Cholecystography

POSITION/PROJECTION: Left Anterior Oblique—Recumbent

ANATOMY: The opacified gall bladder free of superimposition from the spine.

PATIENT/PART POSITION: From the prone position, rotate the patient 15 to 40 degrees to elevate the right side of the body. The left arm is by the side and the right arm is flexed, with the patient resting weight on the elbow. The right leg is flexed, and the patient rests on the right knee to help maintain the position. The head is turned toward the right. Center the image receptor halfway between the spine and the outer edge of the body on the right side of the patient. Using the scout film as a guide, place the image receptor at the level of the gall bladder.

CENTRAL RAY LOCATION/ANGLE: The central ray is directed perpendicular to the center of the image receptor.

NOTES:

BODY PART: Biliary System—Oral Cholecystography

POSITION/PROJECTION: Posteroanterior—Erect

ANATOMY: The opacified gall bladder with any layering of fluids or stratification of stones.

PATIENT/PART POSITION: The patient is placed in the posteroanterior position against an upright grid device. Place a point midway between the spine and the outer edge of the right side of the patient's body to the center of the upright grid device. Using the scout film as a guide, place the image receptor to a point 1 to 3 inches below the gall bladder.

CENTRAL RAY LOCATION/ANGLE: The central ray is directed perpendicular to the center of the image receptor.

NOTES:

BODY PART: Biliary System—Oral Cholecystography

POSITION/PROJECTION: Right Lateral Decubitus

ANATOMY: Used as a supplement to or as a substitute for an image taken in the erect position, this projection demonstrates fluid levels or stone layering without overlying bowel shadows obscuring the opacified gall bladder.

PATIENT/PART POSITION: The patient lies on the right side on a stretcher or table against an upright grid device. The patient's arms should be elevated near the head and the legs placed on top of one another, knees flexed. Center midway between the midsagittal plane and right side of the body, at the level of the gall bladder as determined from the scout film. The bottom edge of film should be below the dependent side of patient.

CENTRAL RAY LOCATION/ANGLE: The central ray is directed perpendicular to the center of the image receptor.

NOTES:

GASTROINTESTINAL SYSTEM

GENERAL TECHNICAL TIPS:
DID YOU
REMEMBER TO?

- use a table pad to provide for the patient's comfort?

- have a pillow and clean linen available for each patient?

- have a compression paddle available?

- have protective aprons and gloves available?

- have the proper type and number of spot films available during fluoroscopy?

- properly identify the patient?

- elicit a history from the patient to include reasons for the exam, any previous conditions, or surgery?

- explain the examination to the patient?

- ask a female patient if she may be pregnant?

- use the ten-day rule in cases of suspected pregnancy?

- introduce the doctor to the patient?

- use a water-soluble iodinated contrast medium in cases of suspected perforations?

- observe the location, size, and shape of the stomach during fluoroscopy?

- properly shield the patient (if possible)?

- collimate to the part?

- have the patient drink continuously for esophageal examinations?

- utilize slightly different positioning based on the patient's bodily habitus?

- follow the departmental protocol regarding the time(s) and amount(s) of barium the patient must ingest during a GI series?

- record the time of administration of the contrast media and utilize time markers on each radiograph?

- position the patient prone to have a barium filled pylorus and supine for an air filled (double contrast)?

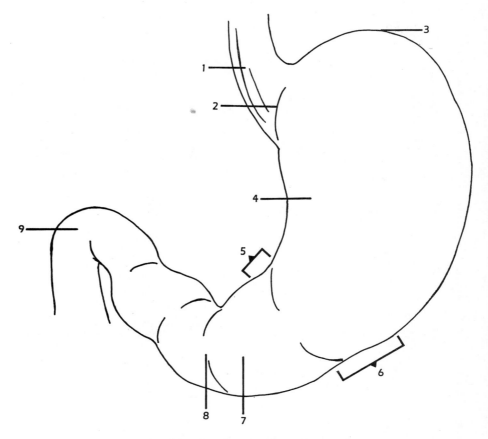

Anterior **A**spect of the **S**tomach

1. Esophagus
2. Cardiac Orifice
3. Fundus
4. Body
5. Lesser Curvature

6. Greater Curvature
7. Pylorus
8. Pyloric Sphincter
9. Duodenum

BODY PART: Gastrointestinal System—Esophagram

POSITION/PROJECTION: Posteroanterior

ANATOMY: The projection will demonstrate the esophagus filled with barium. It may be used to demonstrate strictures, perforations, intraluminal lesions, foreign bodies, esophageal regurgitation, variceals, or hiatal hernia.

PATIENT/PART POSITION: With the patient in the posteroanterior position, center the midsagittal plane to the midline of the table. Place the top of the image receptor at the level of the patient's occlusal plane. The exposure is made while the patient ingests a positive contrast agent.

CENTRAL RAY LOCATION/ANGLE: The central ray is directed perpendicular to the center of the image receptor.

NOTES:

The patient will need to turn his head toward one side in order drink.

BODY PART: Gastrointestinal System—Esophagram

POSITION/PROJECTION: Left Lateral

ANATOMY: An unobstructed projection of the esophagus, filled with barium, in a left lateral position, its shadow projected between the shadows of the spine and mediastinal structures.

PATIENT/PART POSITION: Place the patient in the left lateral position, with the arms drawn in front of or above the head. Center the midaxillary line to the midline of the table. Place the top of the image receptor at the level of the patient's occlusal plane. The exposure is made while the patient ingests a positive contrast agent.

CENTRAL RAY LOCATION/ANGLE: The central ray is directed perpendicular to the midpoint of the image receptor.

NOTES:

BODY PART: Gastrointestinal System—Esophagram

POSITION/PROJECTION: Left Anterior Oblique

ANATOMY: An unobstructed projection of the esophagus, filled with barium, in a left anterior oblique position, its shadow projected between the shadows of the spine and mediastinal structures.

PATIENT/PART POSITION: The patient is placed in a 35- to 40-degree LAO position. Place the left arm by the side and flex the right arm to support the body. Center to a sagittal plane 1 to 2 inches to the right of the spine. Place the top of the image receptor at the level of the patient's occlusal plane. The exposure is made while the patient ingests a positive contrast agent.

CENTRAL RAY LOCATION/ANGLE: The central ray is directed perpendicular to the midpoint of the image receptor.

NOTES:

BODY PART: Gastrointestinal System—Esophagram

POSITION/PROJECTION: Right Anterior Oblique

ANATOMY: An unobstructed projection of the esophagus, filled with barium, in a right anterior oblique position, its shadow projected between the shadows of the spine and mediastinal structures.

PATIENT/PART POSITION: Place the patient in a 35- to 45-degree RAO position. Place the right arm by the side and flex the left arm for support. Center to a sagittal plane 1 to 2 inches to the left of the spine. Place the top of the image receptor at the level of the patient's occlusal plane. The exposure is made while the patient ingest a positive contrast agent.

CENTRAL RAY LOCATION/ANGLE: The central ray is directed perpendicular to the midpoint of the image receptor.

NOTES:

BODY PART: Gastrointestinal System—Gastrointestinal Series

POSITION/PROJECTION: Right Anterior Oblique

ANATOMY: The stomach and the entire duodenal sweep. This projection gives the best image of the pyloric canal and the duodenal bulb in the sthenic type body habitus.

PATIENT/PART POSITION: Start with the patient prone. Instruct the patient to place the right arm at his or her side. Have the patient turn toward the left, using the left forearm and flexed left knee for support. The degree of obliquity depends on the patient's bodily habitus; it will be between 40 and 70 degrees. Bisect the area between the tip of the scapula and the iliac crest and center the image receptor to this point. The stomach can be located at a point midway between the spine and the left side of the body.

CENTRAL RAY LOCATION/ANGLE: Direct the central ray perpendicular to the midpoint of the image receptor.

NOTES:

BODY PART: Gastrointestinal System—Gastrointestinal Series

POSITION/PROJECTION: Posteroanterior

ANATOMY: The pylorus, the duodenal sweep, and the duodenal bulb filled with barium and the fundus filled with air.

PATIENT/PART POSITION: The patient is placed in the prone position on the table, so that the midline of the table coincides with a sagittal plane passing approximately 2 inches to the left of the spine. Center the image receptor to a point midway between the tip of the scapula and the top of the iliac crest.

CENTRAL RAY LOCATION/ANGLE: The central ray is directed perpendicular to the midpoint of the image receptor.

NOTES:

BODY PART: Gastrointestinal System—Gastrointestinal Series

POSITION/PROJECTION: Right Lateral

ANATOMY: The anterior and posterior aspects of the stomach, the pyloric canal, and the duodenal bulb. This affords the best position of the pyloric canal and the duodenal bulb in the hypersthenic body habitus.

PATIENT/PART POSITION: With the patient lying on the right side, center the body to a coronal plane midway between the midaxillary line and the anterior abdomen. Center the image receptor to a point midway between the tip of the scapula and the top of the iliac crest.

CENTRAL RAY LOCATION/ANGLE: The central ray is directed perpendicular to the midpoint of the image receptor.

NOTES:

BODY PART: Gastrointestinal System—Gastrointestinal Series

POSITION/PROJECTION: Left Posterior Oblique

ANATOMY: The stomach and the entire duodenal sweep filled with air; the fundus filled with barium.

PATIENT/PART POSITION: Roll the supine patient 45 degrees toward the left side. Leaving the left arm down on the table, place the right arm across the chest with the right hand resting on the left shoulder. Bend the patient's right leg to help stabilize the position. Center midway between the tip of the scapula and the top of the iliac crest and to the sagittal plane passing midway between the spine and left outer margin of the abdomen.

CENTRAL RAY LOCATION/ANGLE: The central ray is directed perpendicular to the center of the image receptor.

NOTES:

BODY PART: Gastrointestinal System—Gastrointestinal Series

POSITION/PROJECTION: Anteroposterior

ANATOMY: The fundus well filled with barium and the pylorus filled with air. Also demonstrates the retrogastric portion of the duodenum and jejunum.

PATIENT/PART POSITION: With the patient in a supine position, center the midsagittal plane of the body to the center of the table. Place the center of the image receptor approximately 2 to 3 inches above the top of the iliac crest.

CENTRAL RAY LOCATION/ANGLE: The central ray is directed perpendicular to the center of the image receptor.

NOTES:

BODY PART: Gastrointestinal System—Small Bowel Series

POSITION/PROJECTION: Anteroposterior

ANATOMY: The peristaltic function of the digestive tract and detection of any abnormality outlined by the advancing column of contrast material.

PATIENT/PART POSITION: With the patient supine on the table, center the midsagittal plane to the center of the table. For the early films in the series, place the center of the image receptor 2 to 3 inches above the top of the iliac crest. As the exam progresses and the column of contrast material moves from the stomach and proximal portions of the small intestine to the middle and distal portions of the small bowel, adjust the center of the image receptor to coincide with the top of the iliac crest. These films may also be done with the patient in a prone position. All positioning criteria are the same, except that the patient is placed in a prone position on the table.

CENTRAL RAY LOCATION/ANGLE: The central ray is directed perpendicular to the center of the image receptor.

NOTES:

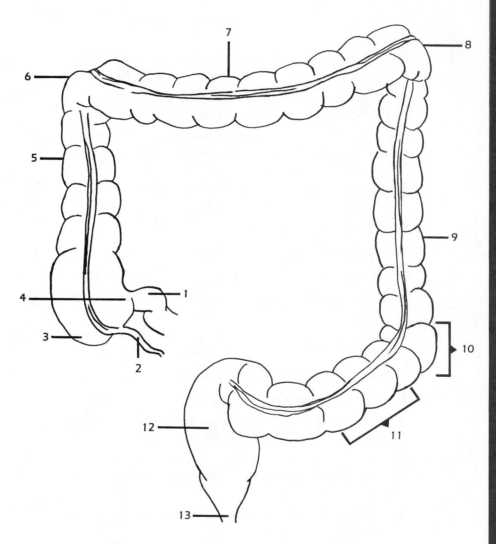

Anterior Aspect of Large Intestine

1. Ileum
2. Vermiform Appendix
3. Cecum
4. Ileocecal Valve
5. Ascending Colon
6. Hepatic Flexure
7. Transverse Colon

8. Splenic Flexure
9. Descending Colon
10. Haustrum
11. Sigmoid Colon
12. Rectum
13. Anus

BARIUM ENEMA

GENERAL TECHNICAL TIPS: DID YOU REMEMBER TO?

■ have lead aprons and gloves available?

■ have the proper type and number of spot films available?

■ have the proper supplies (i.e., gloves, antiseptic solution, incontinent pads, and the like) on hand?

■ check the proper departmental protocol regarding the placement and use of enema tips and retention cuffs?

■ check your hospital's routine regarding double contrast studies (including need for cassette holders, grid cassettes, decubitus sponges, and the like)?

■ check your hospital's procedure for performing barium enemas on colostomy patients?

■ properly identify the patient?

■ ask a female patient if she may be pregnant?

■ use the ten-day rule in cases of suspected pregnancy?

■ elicit a history from the patient to include reasons for the exam, any previous conditions, or surgery?

■ check with the patient regarding the completeness of the preparation for this examination?

■ have the patient void prior to the examination?

■ explain the procedure to the patient?

■ attend to the patient's needs for modesty and comfort as much as possible during this procedure?

■ instruct the patient that deep breathing will alleviate some of the abdominal cramps experienced during the examination?

■ place the patient in a Sim's position for insertion of the enema tip?

■ get assistance whenever resistance is encountered during insertion of the enema tip?

■ check the patient frequently during the evacuation portion of the procedure?

■ properly shield the patient (if possible)?

■ collimate to the part?

BODY PART: Gastrointestinal System—Barium Enema

POSITION/PROJECTION: Anteroposterior

ANATOMY: An anteroposterior projection of the large intestine filled with barium.

PATIENT/PART POSITION: The patient is supine on the table. Center the midsagittal plane to the midline of the table. The center of the image receptor is placed at the level of the iliac crest.

CENTRAL RAY LOCATION/ANGLE: The central ray is directed perpendicular to the midpoint of the image receptor.

NOTES:

BODY PART: Gastrointestinal System—Barium Enema

POSITION/PROJECTION: Anteroposterior Axial

ANATOMY: The sweep of the sigmoid colon, uncoiled and filled with barium.

PATIENT/PART POSITION: The patient is supine on the table, midsagittal plane centered to the midline of the table.

CENTRAL RAY LOCATION/ANGLE: The central ray is directed at a 30- to 35-degree cephalic angle to enter at the level of the symphysis pubis.

NOTES:

BODY PART: Gastrointestinal System—Barium Enema

POSITION/PROJECTION: Right and Left Posterior Obliques

ANATOMY: The left posterior oblique position will demonstrate the hepatic flexure uncoiled and filled with barium, as well as the sigmoid colon. The right posterior oblique position will demonstrate the splenic flexure uncoiled and filled with barium.

PATIENT/PART POSITION: The patient is supine on the table and rotated 45 degrees toward the desired side. Center the horizontal axis of the image receptor to the top of the iliac crest and the long axis of the image receptor to a sagittal plane 1 inch medial to the elevated anterior superior iliac spine.

CENTRAL RAY LOCATION/ANGLE: The central ray is directed perpendicular to the midpoint of the image receptor.

NOTES:

BODY PART: Gastrointestinal System—Barium Enema

POSITION/PROJECTION: Left Lateral

ANATOMY: A profile view of the rectum and sigmoid colon filled with barium.

PATIENT/PART POSITION: The patient is put in a true left lateral position, flexing the hips and knees to help maintain the position. Center the patient by placing the coronal plane 2 inches posterior to the midaxillary line in the center of the table. The image receptor should be centered to a point about 2 inches superior to the symphysis publis.

CENTRAL RAY LOCATION/ANGLE: The central ray is directed perpendicular to the center of the image receptor.

NOTES:

BODY PART: Gastrointestinal System—Barium Enema—Double Contrast

POSITION/PROJECTION: Posteroanterior and Anteroposterior with Table Tilt

ANATOMY: The large intestine, demonstrated by the administration of both positive and negative contrast agents. Internal growths such as polyps are well demonstrated.

PATIENT/PART POSITION: The patient is supine (for the AP) or prone (for the PA) on the table. Table may be tilted, head down, 10 to 15 degrees. Center the midsagittal plane to the midline of the table. The center of the image receptor is placed at the level of the iliac crest.

CENTRAL RAY LOCATION/ANGLE: The central ray is directed perpendicular to the midpoint of the image receptor.

NOTES:

BODY PART: Gastrointestinal System—Barium Enema—Double Contrast

POSITION/PROJECTION: Lateral Decubitus—Right and Left

ANATOMY: The large intestine demonstrated by the administration of both positive and negative contrast agents. Right lateral decubitus: medial wall of the ascending colon, lateral wall of descending colon, splenic flexure; all these areas will be air filled. Left lateral decubitus: lateral wall of the ascending colon, medial wall of descending colon, hepatic flexure; all these areas will be air filled. Internal growths such as polyps are well demonstrated.

PATIENT/PART POSITION: The patient is placed in a lateral recumbent position with knees flexed and legs resting together. The arms are raised above the head, elbows flexed. Center the midsagittal plane to the midline of the erect Bucky or grid holder. The center of the image receptor is placed at the level of the iliac crests.

CENTRAL RAY LOCATION/ANGLE: The central ray is directed perpendicular to the midpoint of the image receptor.

NOTES:

In order to demonstrate air/fluid levels, the central ray **MUST** be parallel to the floor.

PART

6

Spinal Column

Cervical Spine 176

Thoracic Spine 184

Lumbosacral Spine 190

Sacrum and Coccyx 198

Sacroiliac Joints 203

SPINAL COLUMN

GENERAL TECHNICAL TIPS: DID YOU REMEMBER TO?

■ properly identify the patient?

■ ask a female patient if she may be pregnant?

■ use the ten-day rule in cases of suspected pregnancy?

■ assess the patient's injury and/or get a thorough history before moving the patient or placing the patient in any position?

■ remove and secure any opaque objects from the field of interest?

■ utilize the anode-heel effect appropriately?

■ respect the patient's modesty by providing linen to properly cover the patient?

■ properly shield the patient (if possible)?

■ use positioning sponges to assist in maintaining the patient's position?

■ collimate to the part?

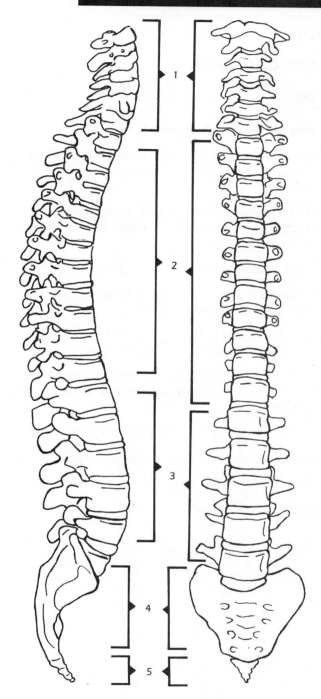

Lateral Aspect   Anterior Aspect

Vertebral Column

1. Cervical   **4.** Sacrum
2. Thoracic   **5.** Coccyx
3. Lumbar

CERVICAL SPINE

GENERAL TECHNICAL TIPS: DID YOU REMEMBER TO?

- ■ properly identify the patient?

- ■ refrain from moving **ANY** trauma patient until a cross-table lateral film has been done and checked by a radiologist?

- ■ elicit a history from each patient and assess the patient's condition prior to performing routine views of the cervical spine?

- ■ ask a female patient if she may be pregnant?

- ■ remove and secure all necklaces, earrings, bobbi pins, and other radiopaque objects?

- ■ raise the patient's chin on the AP to avoid superimposition of the mandible and cervical spine?

- ■ have the patient hold equally weighted sandbags in the lateral view(s) to clearly demonstrate the lower cervical vertebrae?

- ■ expose all views while the patient is in expiration?

- ■ check all exposure factors, especially exposure time?

- ■ properly shield the patient?

- ■ collimate to the part?

1. **S**uperior **A**spect of **A**tlas
   A. Foramen for Vertebral Artery and Vein
   B. Anterior Arch
   C. Superior Articular Facet
   D. Transverse Process
   E. Posterior Arch

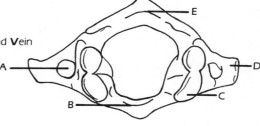

2. **L**ateral **A**spect of **A**xis
   A. Body
   B. Superior Articular Process
   C. Transverse Process
   D. Inferior Articular Process
   E. Spinous Process
   F. Odontoid Process

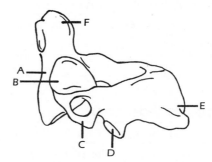

3. **A**nterior **A**spect of **A**xis
   A. Body
   B. Superior Articular Process
   C. Transverse Process
   D. Inferior Articular Process
   E. Odontoid Process

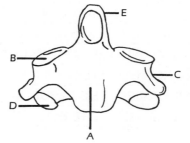

4. **S**uperior **A**spect of **C**ervical **V**ertebrae
   A. Spinous Process
   B. Lamina
   C. Superior Articular Process
   D. Pedicle
   E. Transverse Foramen
   F. Transverse Process

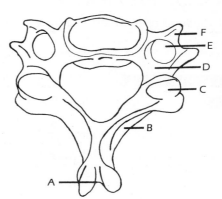

Cervical **V**ertebrae

BODY PART: Cervical Spine

POSITION/PROJECTION: Lateral

ANATOMY: A lateral projection of the cervical vertebrae, one through seven, including the bodies, interspaces, spinous processes, articular pillars; and the the articular facets of vertebrae three through seven.

PATIENT/PART POSITION: The patient is seated or standing erect with the shoulder against the upright Bucky. Set the coronal plane passing through the mastoid tips to the center of the upright Bucky. Elevate the chin and stick out the jaw so that the mandible does not superimpose over the spine. The image receptor is placed so that the top of the film is at the top of the patient's ear. Lateral views may be done with the neck in extension, flexion, and a neutral position. **FOR A PATIENT WHO HAS SUSTAINED A SUSPECTED SEVERE INJURY TO THE NECK, THE LATERAL VIEW SHOULD BE DONE FIRST ON THE STRETCHER OR BED. THE RESULTING FILM MUST BE CHECKED BY A PHYSICIAN BEFORE THE PATIENT IS MOVED.**

CENTRAL RAY LOCATION/ANGLE: The central ray is directed perpendicular to enter at the level of the fourth cervical vertebra.

NOTES:

When the lower cervical vertebrae and interspaces are not clearly visualized, a lateral (Swimmer's)—Twining method must be performed.

BODY PART: Cervicothoracic Spine

POSITION/PROJECTION: Lateral (Swimmer's)—Twining Method

ANATOMY: A lateral projection of the lower cervical vertebral bodies, cervical intervertebral disk spaces, upper thoracic vertebral bodies, thoracic intervertebral disk spaces, and posterior structures.

PATIENT/PART POSITION: The patient is lateral recumbent or upright, with the midaxillary plane aligned with the midline of the table or upright Bucky. The arm nearest the image receptor is elevated, and the shoulder on this side is moved anterior. The hand is placed on or near the patient's head. The opposite arm is placed down and the shoulder on this side is moved posterior. The spine is placed in a true lateral position. The image receptor is centered to the second thoracic vertebra, which lies ¾ inch above the suprasternal notch.

CENTRAL RAY LOCATION/ANGLE: The central ray is directed perpendicular to the midpoint of the image receptor.

NOTES:

BODY PART: Cervical Spine

POSITION/PROJECTION: Anteroposterior of the Atlas and Axis

ANATOMY: The atlas and axis through the open mouth of the patient.

PATIENT/PART POSITION: Place the patient supine or erect AP, so that the midsagittal plane is centered to the midline of the table or erect Bucky. With the patient's mouth open, adjust the head so that a line from the lower edge of the upper incisors and tip of the mastoids is perpendicular to the film. Place the center of the image receptor in line with the center of the patient's open mouth.

CENTRAL RAY LOCATION/ANGLE: The central ray is directed perpendicular to the midpoint of the image receptor.

NOTES:

BODY PART: Cervical Spine

POSITION/PROJECTION: Anteroposterior of Cervical Vertebrae Three to Seven

ANATOMY: The bodies of cervical vertebrae three through seven, thoracic vertebrae one and two; the interpediculate spaces, transverse and articulate processes, and the intervertebral disk spaces.

PATIENT/PART POSITION: The patient may be either supine or erect, with the midsagittal plane of the body centered to the midline of the table or upright Bucky. The patient's head is adjusted with the chin slightly raised so that the occlusal plane and the mastoid tip are perpendicular to the image receptor.

CENTRAL RAY LOCATION/ANGLE: The central ray is directed 15 to 20 degrees cephalic to enter at the level of the fourth cervical vertebra.

NOTES:

BODY PART: Cervical Spine

POSITION/PROJECTION: Right and Left Posterior Obliques, Right and Left Anterior Obliques

ANATOMY: An oblique projection of the intervertebral foramina, pedicles, and bodies of the cervical spine. The right posterior and left posterior oblique positions demonstrate the foramina and pedicles farthest from the film; the right anterior and left anterior oblique positions demonstrate the foramina and pedicles closest to the film.

PATIENT/PART POSITION: The patient is recumbent or erect and obliqued 45 degrees. Center the midline of the cervical spine to the midline of the image receptor. For anterior obliques, the head is rotated laterally to maintain proper rotation of the spine. For posterior obliques, both the head and body are placed in a 45-degree oblique position. The image receptor is centered to the level of the third to fourth cervical vertebrae.

CENTRAL RAY LOCATION/ANGLE: The central ray is directed 15 to 20 degrees cephalad for the right and left posterior obliques, and 15 to 20 degrees caudad for the right and left anterior obliques.

NOTES:

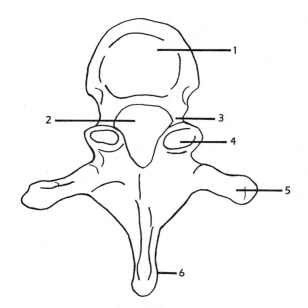

Superior **A**spect

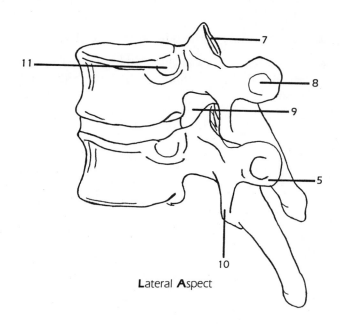

Lateral **A**spect

Thoracic **V**ertebrae

1. **B**ody
2. **V**ertebral **C**anal
3. **P**edicle
4. **A**rticular **F**acet

5. **T**ransverse **P**rocess
6. **S**pinous **P**rocess
7. **S**uperior **A**rticular **P**rocess
8. **F**acet for **T**ubercle of **R**ib

9. **I**ntervertebral **F**oramen
10. **I**nferior **A**rticular **P**rocess
11. **A**rticular **F**acet for **H**ead of **R**ib

THORACIC SPINE

GENERAL TECHNICAL TIPS:
DID YOU
REMEMBER TO?

- properly identify the patient?

- ask a female patient if she may be pregnant?

- use the ten-day rule in cases of suspected pregnancy?

- properly shield the patient?

- collimate to the part?

- properly utilize the anode-heel effect?

- place the patient's arms above the head in the AP to reduce the kyphosis of the thoracic spine?

- support the patient's waist when positioning the lateral, to insure that the spine remains parallel to the film?

- place a lead blocker or lead glove behind the patient's back to absorb excess radiation when exposing the lateral view?

- use a breathing technique on the lateral view?

- use the Swimmer's position when it is necessary to visualize the upper thoracic vertebrae in the lateral position?

BODY PART: Thoracic Spine

POSITION/PROJECTION: Anteroposterior

ANATOMY: An anteroposterior projection of thoracic vertebrae one through twelve, including the bodies, interspaces, and the surrounding structures.

PATIENT/PART POSITION: With the patient supine, knees flexed, and a small pillow under the head (to minimize curvature of spine), center the midsagittal plane to the midline of the table. Place the image receptor so that its upper edge is 1 to 2 inches above the top of the shoulder.

CENTRAL RAY LOCATION/ANGLE: The central ray is directed perpendicular to enter at the level of the sixth thoracic vertebra.

NOTES:

BODY PART: Thoracic Spine

POSITION/PROJECTION: Lateral

ANATOMY: A lateral projection of the twelve thoracic vertebrae including the bodies, the interspaces, the intervertebral foramina, and the lower spinous processes.

PATIENT/PART POSITION: The patient is lying on the left side with a support under the head, knees flexed, and a support under the side to place the spine parallel with the film. The midaxillary line is centered to the midline of the table. The image receptor is placed so the upper border is 1 to 2 inches above the top of the shoulder.

CENTRAL RAY LOCATION/ANGLE: The central ray is directed perpendicular to enter at the level of the sixth thoracic vertebra.

NOTES:

BODY PART: Cervicothoracic Spine

POSITION/PROJECTION: Swimmer's Lateral—Twining Method

ANATOMY: A lateral projection of the lower cervical vertebral bodies, cervical intervertebral disk spaces, upper thoracic vertebral bodies, thoracic intervertebral disk spaces, and posterior structures.

PATIENT/PART POSITION: The patient is lateral recumbent or upright, with the midaxillary plane aligned with the midline of the table or upright Bucky. The arm nearest the image receptor is elevated and the shoulder on this side is moved anterior. The hand is placed on or near the patient's head. The opposite arm is placed down and the shoulder on this side is moved posterior. The spine is placed in a true lateral position. The image receptor is centered to the second thoracic vertebra, which lies ¾ inch above the suprasternal notch.

CENTRAL RAY LOCATION/ANGLE: The central ray is directed perpendicular to the midpoint of the image receptor.

NOTES:

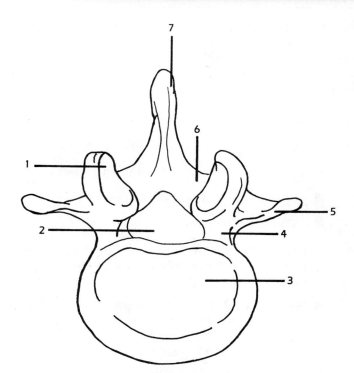

Superior **A**spect

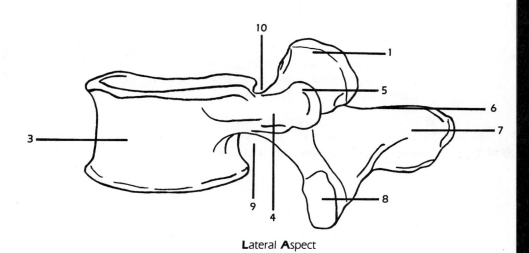

Lateral **A**spect

Lumbar **V**ertebra

1. **S**uperior **A**rticular **P**rocess   **5.** **T**ransverse **P**rocess   **8.** **I**nferior **A**rticular **P**rocess
2. **V**ertebral **F**oramen   **6.** **L**amina   **9.** **I**nferior **V**ertebral **N**otch
3. **B**ody   **7.** **S**pinous **P**rocess   **10.** **S**uperior **V**ertebral **N**otch
4. **P**edicle

LUMBOSACRAL SPINE

GENERAL TECHNICAL TIPS:
DID YOU
REMEMBER TO?

■ properly identify the patient?

■ ask a female patient if she may be pregnant?

■ use the ten-day rule in cases of suspected pregnancy?

■ properly shield the patient (if possible)?

■ collimate to the part?

■ respect the patient's modesty by properly covering the patient when positioning for the various views of the lumber spine?

■ bend the patient's knees and place the feet flat on the table to reduce the normal lumbar lordosis (and make the patient with back spasms more comfortable) while performing the AP position?

■ use sponges to support the patient when performing oblique positions of the lumbar vertebrae?

■ support the patient's waist to insure that the spine remains parallel to the image receptor when positioning for the lateral?

■ place a lead blocker or lead glove behind the patient's back to absorb excess radiation when exposing the lateral view?

■ angle 5 to 8 degrees caudal for the spot lateral of L5–S1, when you are unable to maintain a parallel relationship between the spine and image receptor?

BODY PART: Lumbosacral Spine

POSITION/PROJECTION: Anteroposterior

ANATOMY: An AP projection of the lumbar bodies, the interpediculate spaces, the intervertebral disk spaces, the laminae, and the spinous and transverse processes.

PATIENT/PART POSITION: Center the midsagittal plane of the body to the midline of the table. Flex the hips and knees enough to place the back in firm contact with the table in order to delineate the intervertebral disk spaces. Center the image receptor at a point ½ to 1 inch above the iliac crests.

CENTRAL RAY LOCATION/ANGLE: Direct the central ray perpendicular to the midpoint of the image receptor.

NOTES:

BODY PART: Lumbosacral Spine

POSITION/PROJECTION: Anteroposterior Axial

ANATOMY: The lumbosacral area and sacroiliac joints.

PATIENT/PART POSITION: With the patient supine and the lower extremities extended, direct the central ray cephalad 30 to 35 degrees to enter at the level of the anterior superior iliac spines. Center the midsagittal plane to the midline of the table.

CENTRAL RAY LOCATION/ANGLE: Direct the central ray as noted above to the midpoint of the image receptor.

NOTES:

BODY PART: Lumbosacral Spine

POSITION/PROJECTION: Right and Left Posterior Obliques

ANATOMY: The articular facets of the side nearest the film.

PATIENT/PART POSITION: Have the patient turn from the supine position to a 45-degree oblique position. Center the spine to the midline of the table by centering to a sagittal plane 1½ inches medial to the anterior superior iliac spine of the elevated side. Center the image receptor ½ to 1 inch above the top of the iliac crest.

CENTRAL RAY LOCATION/ANGLE: Direct the central ray perpendicular to the midpoint of the image receptor.

NOTES:

BODY PART: Lumbosacral Spine

POSITION/PROJECTION: Lateral

ANATOMY: A lateral projection of the lumbar bodies and interspaces, the spinous processes, the lumbosacral junction, and the sacrum and coccyx.

PATIENT/PART POSITION: Have the patient turn on the left side and flex the hips and knees to a comfortable position. Center the midaxillary line of the body to the midline of the table. Center the image receptor ½ to 1 inch above the level of the iliac crest.

CENTRAL RAY LOCATION/ANGLE: Direct the central ray perpendicular to the midpoint of the image receptor.

NOTES:

BODY PART: Lumbosacral Spine

POSITION/PROJECTION: Localized Lateral (L5–S1 Spot)

ANATOMY: A lateral projection of the lumbosacral joint, the lower one or two lumbar vertebrae, and the upper sacrum.

PATIENT/PART POSITION: With the patient in the same position as the lateral projection, direct the central ray caudally 5 to 8 degrees.* The central ray enters midway between the level of the iliac crest and the anterior superior iliac spine. Align the patient's body so that a coronal plane 1½ inches posterior to the midaxillary line is centered to the midline of the table.

CENTRAL RAY LOCATION/ANGLE: Direct the central ray at the previously listed angle to the midpoint of the image receptor.

NOTES:

*Angulation is necessary only when a parallel relationship cannot be maintained between the spine and the image receptor.

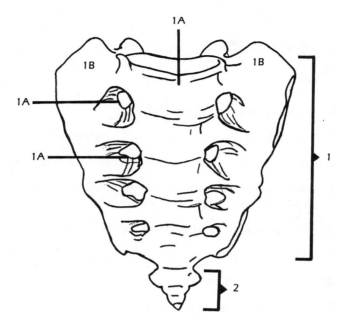

Anterior **A**spect

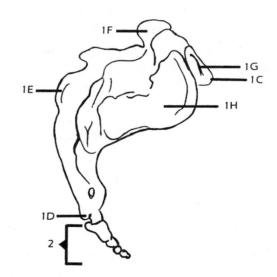

Lateral **A**spect

Sacrum and **C**occyx

1. Sacrum
  A. Anterior **S**acral **F**oramina
  B. Ala
  C. Promontory
  D. Cornu
  E. Medial **S**acral **C**rest
  F. Articular **P**rocess
  G. Body
  H. Auricular **S**urface

2. Coccyx

SACRUM AND COCCYX

GENERAL TECHNICAL TIPS: DID YOU REMEMBER TO?

■ properly identify the patient?

■ ask a female patient if she may be pregnant?

■ use the ten-day rule in cases of suspected pregnancy?

■ assess the patient's injury before having the patient lie supine on the table?

■ have the patient void prior to the exam?

■ properly shield the patient (if possible)?

■ collimate to the part?

■ angle 15 degrees cephalad for the AP sacrum?

■ angle 10 degrees caudally for the AP coccyx?

■ use decreased exposure factors for a lateral coccyx compared to those used for a lateral sacrum?

■ use lead blockers or lead gloves behind the patient to absorb excess radiation when performing the lateral positions?

BODY PART: Sacrum

POSITION/PROJECTION: Anteroposterior

ANATOMY: An anteroposterior projection of the sacrum free of any superimposition.

PATIENT/PART POSITION: The patient is supine with the midsagittal plane centered to the midline of the table.

CENTRAL RAY LOCATION/ANGLE: The central ray is directed 15 degrees cephalad, to enter at a point halfway between the symphysis pubis and the anterior superior iliac spines, and centered to the midpoint of the image receptor.

NOTES:

BODY PART: Sacrum

POSITION/PROJECTION: Lateral

ANATOMY: A lateral projection of the entire sacrum.

PATIENT/PART POSITION: The patient is lying on the left side with the knees and hips flexed. The body is centered to the midline of the table by aligning a coronal plane 3 inches posterior to the midaxillary line or by aligning a coronal plane 2 inches anterior to the posterior surface of the sacrum. Center the image receptor to the level of the anterior superior iliac spines.

CENTRAL RAY LOCATION/ANGLE: The central ray is directed perpendicular to the midpoint of the image receptor.

NOTES:

BODY PART: Coccyx

POSITION/PROJECTION: Anteroposterior

ANATOMY: A frontal projection of the coccyx without superimposition of the symphysis pubis.

PATIENT/PART POSITION: The patient is supine with the midsagittal plane centered to the midline of the table.

CENTRAL RAY LOCATION/ANGLE: The central ray is directed 10 degrees caudad to enter at a point 1½ inches superior to the symphysis pubis and centered to the midpoint of the image receptor.

NOTES:

Close collimation is essential for increased visibility of this structure.

BODY PART: Coccyx

POSITION/PROJECTION: Lateral

ANATOMY: A lateral projection of the entire coccyx.

PATIENT/PART POSITION: The patient is lying on the left side with the knees and hips flexed. The long axis of the coccyx is centered to the midline of the table. Center superior to the tip of the coccyx (mid-coccyx).

CENTRAL RAY LOCATION/ANGLE: The central ray is directed perpendicular, to enter the mid-coccyx region.

NOTES:

Close collimation is essential for increased visibility of this structure.

BODY PART: Sacroiliac Joints

POSITION/PROJECTION: Right and Left Posterior Obliques

ANATOMY: The sacroiliac joint farthest from the film in a profile projection.

PATIENT/PART POSITION: From a supine position, rotate the patient to a 25- to 30-degree oblique position. The patient is centered to a coronal plane 1 inch medial to the anterior superior iliac spine of the elevated joint.

CENTRAL RAY LOCATION/ANGLE: The central ray is directed perpendicular to the anterior superior iliac spine of the elevated side.

NOTES:

PART
7

CRANIAL AND FACIAL BONES

Skull 213

Optic Foramen 221

Facial Bones 225

Nasal Bones 231

Zygomatic Arches 235

Mandible 239

Temporomandibular Joints 245

Paranasal Sinuses 249

Temporal Bone—Mastoids 255

Temporal Bone—Petrous Portion 261

CRANIAL AND FACIAL BONES

GENERAL TECHNICAL TIPS:
DID YOU
REMEMBER TO?

■ properly identify the patient?

■ ask a female patient if she might be pregnant?

■ use the ten-day rule in cases of suspected pregnancy?

■ remove all radiopaque objects (including dentures) from the head and neck?

■ assess any patients who may have a cranial shape other than mesocephalic and adjust your positioning appropriately?

■ position the patient from a sitting or standing position whenever possible?

■ use the proper markers on each position performed?

■ utilize positioning and immobilizing devices whenever necessary?

■ use all surface landmarks and planes required by the various positions?

■ utilize cranial angulators to check positioning?

■ check your source-to-image distance?

■ properly shield the patient?

■ place the patient in position last so as to decrease any discomfort?

■ collimate to the part?

■ suspend respiration for all views?

■ use the small focal spot?

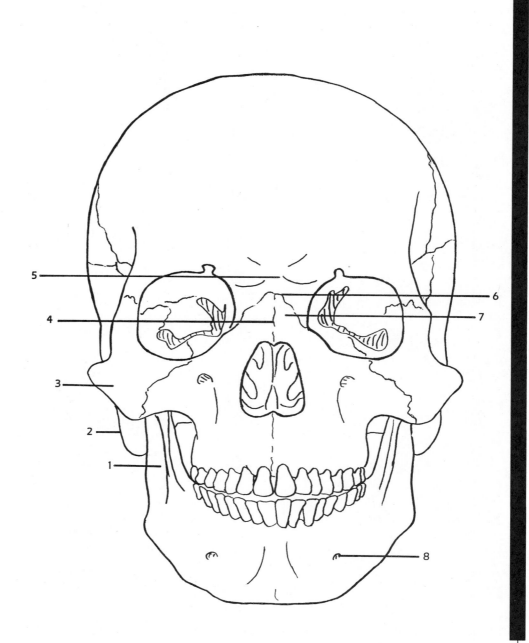

Anterior Aspect of Skull

1. Ramus of Mandible
2. Mastoid Process
3. Zygomatic Arch
4. Internasal Suture

5. Glabella
6. Nasion
7. Nasal Bones
8. Mental Foramen

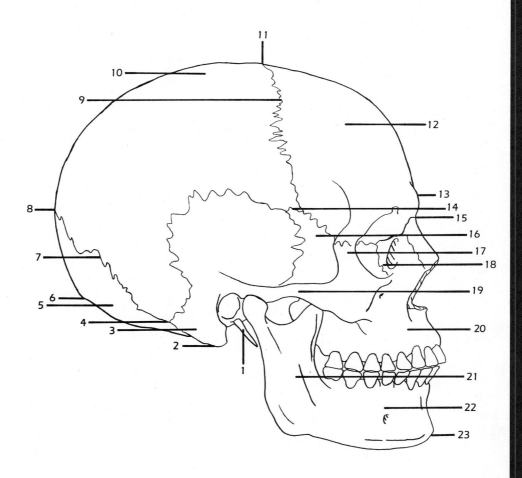

Lateral Aspect of Skull

1. Temporal Styloid Process
2. Mastoid Process
3. Temporal Bone
4. Asterion
5. Occipital Bone
6. External Occipital Protuberance
7. Lambdoidal Suture
8. Lambda

9. Coronal Suture
10. Parietal Bone
11. Bregma
12. Frontal Bone
13. Glabella
14. Pterion
15. Nasion
16. Sphenoid Bone

17. Zygomatic Bone
18. Ethmoid Bone
19. Zygomatic Arch
20. Maxilla
21. Ramus of Mandible
22. Body of Mandible
23. Mental Protuberance

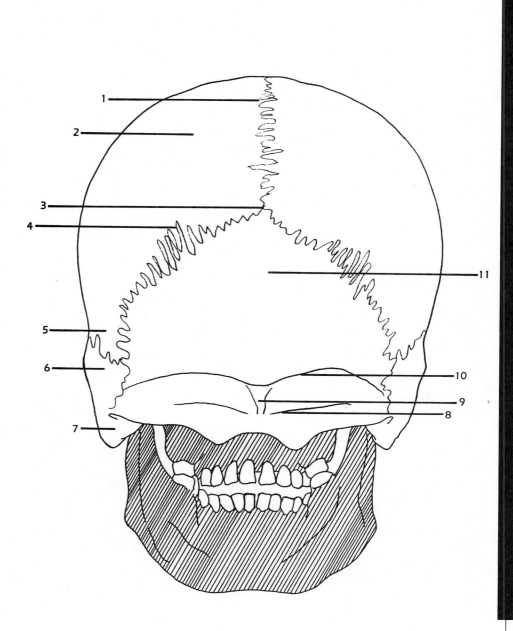

Posterior Aspect of Skull

1. Sagittal Suture
2. Parietal Bone
3. Lambda
4. Lambdoidal Suture
5. Asterion
6. Temporal Bone
7. Mastoid Process
8. Inferior Nuchal Line
9. Inion or External Occipital Protuberance
10. Superior Nuchal Line
11. Occipital Bone

SKULL

GENERAL TECHNICAL TIPS: DID YOU REMEMBER TO?

- ■ properly identify the patient?

- ■ properly shield the patient?

- ■ collimate to the part?

- ■ use the Haas method, in lieu of the Grashey method, for patients with severe kyphosis?

- ■ use a sitting or standing position to perform the Schuller method whenever possible?

BODY PART: Skull

POSITION/PROJECTION: Posteroanterior

ANATOMY: A posteroanterior projection of the anterior wall of the cranium, the frontal sinuses, the crista galli, and the ethmoid sinuses. The petrous ridges will completely fill the orbit.

PATIENT/PART POSITION: The patient is placed prone on the table or facing the upright grid device with the forehead and nose placed against the table or upright Bucky. The midsagittal and orbitomeatal lines are placed perpendicular to the image receptor. The top of the image receptor is placed 1½ inches above the vertex.

CENTRAL RAY LOCATION/ANGLE: The central ray is directed perpendicular to the nasion.

NOTES:

BODY PART: Skull

POSITION/PROJECTION: Posteroanterior—Caldwell Method

ANATOMY: A posteroanterior projection of the frontal bone, the greater and lesser wings of the sphenoid, the frontal and ethmoid sinuses, the crista galli, and the upper two-thirds of the orbits. The petrous ridges will be projected in the lower third of the orbits.

PATIENT/PART POSITION: The patient is placed prone on the table or facing the upright grid device, with the forehead and nose placed against the table or upright Bucky. The midsagittal and orbitomeatal lines are placed perpendicular to the image receptor. The top of the image receptor is placed 1½ inches above the vertex.

CENTRAL RAY LOCATION/ANGLE: The central ray is directed 15 degrees caudally to pass through the nasion.

NOTES:

BODY PART: Skull

POSITION/PROJECTION: Anteroposterior Axial—Grashey Method

ANATOMY: A PA axial projection of the occipital region of the cranium, a symmetrical view of the petrous pyramids, and the dorsum sellae within the shadow of the foramen magnum. This view is used for obese patients and patients who cannot be adjusted into a Grashey method position.

PATIENT/PART POSITION: The patient is prone on the table with the nose and forehead down. Adjust the midsagittal plane and the orbitomeatal line perpendicular to the image receptor.

CENTRAL RAY LOCATION/ANGLE: The central ray is directed caudally to pass through the foramen magnum at a 30 degree angle.

*Some patients may require that the infraorbitomeatal line be placed perpendicular to the image receptor. In these cases, a 37-degree caudal angle will be used.

NOTES:

BODY PART: Skull

POSITION/PROJECTION: Posteroanterior Axial—Haas Method (Reverse Grashey)

ANATOMY: A PA axial projection of the occipital region of the cranium, a symmetrical view of the petrous pyramids, and the dorsum sellae within the shadow of the foramen magnum. This view is used for obese patients and patients who cannot be adjusted into a Townes method position.

PATIENT/PART POSITION: The patient is prone on the table with the nose and forehead down. Adjust the midsagittal plane and the orbitomeatal line perpendicular to the image receptor.

CENTRAL RAY LOCATION/ANGLE: The central ray is directed 25 degrees cephalic and enters at a point 1½ inches below the inion. The central ray will exit 1½ inches above the nasion.

TUBE

25°

NOTES:

BODY PART: Skull

POSITION/PROJECTION: Lateral

ANATOMY: A lateral projection of the superimposed parietal bones, the sella turcica, the sphenoid sinus, and the anterior and posterior clinoid processes.

PATIENT/PART POSITION: The patient is either prone or facing the upright Bucky. The head is adjusted to a lateral position. If the patient is on the table, the semi-prone position is required. The midsagittal plane is placed parallel and the interpupillary line placed perpendicular to the table or upright Bucky. The top of the image receptor is placed 1½ inches above the vertex.

CENTRAL RAY LOCATION/ANGLE: The central ray is directed perpendicular to the image receptor. It enters a point ¾ inch anterior and superior to the external auditory meatus (EAM).

NOTES:

BODY PART: Skull

POSITION/PROJECTION: Submentovertical—Schuller Method

ANATOMY: A full basal projection of the cranium including the petrosae, the mastoid processes, the petrous pyramids, the foramina ovale and spinosum, the sphenoid sinus, the mandible, the foramen magnum, the odontoid process, and the entire atlas.

PATIENT/PART POSITION: The patient is either sitting, with the vertex resting against the upright Bucky, or supine on the table, with pillows or sponges under the shoulders to assist in hyperextending the head and neck. The infraorbitomeatal line is adjusted as parallel as possible to the image receptor. The vertex of the head and the midsagittal plane is adjusted so it is perpendicular to the image receptor.

CENTRAL RAY LOCATION/ANGLE: The central ray is directed perpendicular to the infraorbitomeatal line, entering midway between the mandibular angles. The degree of angulation of the central ray will depend on the degree of hyperextension of the patient's head and neck.

NOTES:

BODY PART: Skull

POSITION/PROJECTION: Verticosubmental—Schuller Method

ANATOMY: Demonstrates approximately the same structures as the submentovertical but does demonstrate the sphenoid sinuses and anterior cranial base more clearly.

PATIENT/PART POSITION: For a VSM, the patient is prone, with the head resting on the chin and midsagittal plane perpendicular to the image receptor. Place the infraorbitomeatal line as close to parallel to the image receptor as possible.

CENTRAL RAY LOCATION/ANGLE: The central ray is directed through the sella turcica, perpendicular to the infraorbitomeatal line. The central ray passes through a point ¾ inch anterior to the EAM.

NOTES:

OPTIC FORAMEN

GENERAL TECHNICAL TIPS:
DID YOU
REMEMBER TO?

- ■ properly identify the patient?

- ■ properly shield the patient?

- ■ collimate to the part?

- ■ use an extension cone, if available?

- ■ use a small focal spot?

- ■ do both sides and correctly mark each film?

BODY PART: Optic Foramen

POSITION/PROJECTION: Parieto-Orbital Projection—Rhese Method

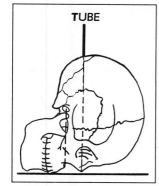

ANATOMY: A cross-sectional projection of the optic canal in the lower outer quadrant of the orbital shadow.

PATIENT/PART POSITION: Center the midsagittal plane of the body to the midline of the image receptor. Rotate the head so that the midsagittal plane forms an angle of 53 degrees with the horizontal. Rest the head on the chin, cheek, and nose. Place the acanthiomeatal line perpendicular to the table and center the image receptor to the dependent orbit.

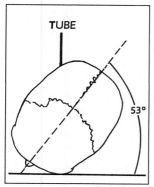

CENTRAL RAY LOCATION/ANGLE: The central ray is directed perpendicular to the midpoint of the image receptor.

NOTES:

This position may also be performed with the patient in a supine or AP position. This variation requires that the uppermost orbit be centered. All other positioning criteria remain the same.

FACIAL BONES

GENERAL TECHNICAL TIPS: DID YOU REMEMBER TO?

- properly identify the patient?

- use the supine positioning for this exam if the patient is unable to maintain the prone position and/or for the comfort of a patient with facial injuries?

- properly shield the patient?

- collimate to the part?

- use an extension cone, if available?

- use a small focal spot?

- check the mentomeatal line for correct flexion in the Waters method position?

- check the interpupillary line when positioning the lateral?

BODY PART: Facial Bones

POSITION/PROJECTION: Posteroanterior—Caldwell Method

ANATOMY: A posteroanterior projection of the frontal bone, the greater and lesser wings of the sphenoid, the frontal and ethmoid sinuses, the crista galli, and the upper two-thirds of the orbits. The petrous ridges will be projected in the lower third of the orbits.

PATIENT/PART POSITION: The patient is placed prone on the table or facing the upright grid device with the forehead and nose placed against the table or upright Bucky. The midsagittal and orbitomeatal lines are placed perpendicular to the image receptor.

CENTRAL RAY LOCATION/ANGLE: The central ray is directed 15 degrees caudally to pass through the nasion.

NOTES:

BODY PART: Facial Bones

POSITION/PROJECTION: Parietoacanthial—Waters Method

ANATOMY: An oblique frontal projection of the facial bones—primarily the orbits, the zygomatic bones, the zygomatic arches, the maxillae, and the maxillary sinuses.

PATIENT/PART POSITION: Center the midsagittal plane of the patient's head to the midline of the table, resting the head on the tip of the extended chin. The midsagittal plane is perpendicular to the image receptor. Adjust the flexion of the head so that the orbitomeatal line forms an angle of 37 degrees with the plane of the image receptor.

CENTRAL RAY LOCATION/ANGLE: The central ray is directed perpendicular to the image receptor to exit at the acanthion.

NOTES:

BODY PART: Facial Bones

POSITION/PROJECTION: Lateral

ANATOMY: The right and left halves of the facial bones superimposed.

PATIENT/PART POSITION: The patient is placed in a lateral skull position.

CENTRAL RAY LOCATION/ANGLE: The central ray is directed perpendicular to the midpoint of the image receptor ½ inch posterior to the outer canthus and at the level of the zygoma.

NOTES:

NASAL BONES

GENERAL TECHNICAL TIPS: DID YOU REMEMBER TO?

- properly identify the patient?
- properly shield the patient?
- collimate to the part?
- use an extension cone, if available?
- use a small focal spot?
- check that the mentomeatal line is perpendicular in the Waters method positon?

BODY PART: Nasal Bones

POSITION/PROJECTION: Lateral

ANATOMY: A lateral projection of the nasal bones and soft tissue structures of the nose on the side nearer the image receptor.

PATIENT/PART POSITION: Adjust the head so that the patient is in a true lateral skull position. Place the image receptor beneath the patient's head, centered to the bridge of the nose. This is a nongrid examination.

CENTRAL RAY LOCATION/ANGLE: The central ray is directed perpendicular to the bridge of the nose to a point ¾ inch below the nasion.

NOTES:

BODY PART: Nasal Bones

POSITION/PROJECTION: Parietoacanthial—Waters Method

ANATOMY: An oblique frontal projection of the facial bones—primarily the orbits, the zygomatic bones, the zygomatic arches, the maxillae, and the maxillary sinuses.

PATIENT/PART POSITION: Center the midsagittal plane of the patient's head to the midline of the table, resting the head on the tip of the extended chin. The midsagittal plane is perpendicular to the image receptor. Adjust the flexion of the head so that the orbitomeatal line forms an angle of 37 degrees with the plane of the image receptor.

CENTRAL RAY LOCATION/ANGLE: The central ray is directed perpendicular to the image receptor to exit at the acanthion.

NOTES:

ZYGOMATIC ARCHES

GENERAL TECHNICAL TIPS:
DID YOU
REMEMBER TO?

- properly identify the patient?
- properly shield the patient?
- collimate to the part?
- use an extension cone, if available?
- use a small focal spot?
- perform the axial projection with the patient in a sitting or standing position, if possible?

BODY PART: Zygomatic Arches

POSITION/PROJECTION: Axial—Submentovertical Projection

ANATOMY: A symmetrical axial view of the zygomatic arches projected free of superimposed structures.

PATIENT/PART POSITION: Center the midsagittal plane of the patient's body to the midline of the table. Rest the head on the vertex, extending the head and neck completely, so that the infraorbitomeatal line is as parallel as possible to the plane of the image receptor. Adjust the head so that the midsagittal plane is perpendicular to the image receptor.

CENTRAL RAY LOCATION/ANGLE: The central ray is directed perpendicular to the infraorbitomeatal line and centered midway between the zygomatic arches. The central ray will pass through a coronal plane lying 1 inch posterior to the outer canthi.

NOTES:

This examination may be accomplished as a grid or nongrid examination.

BODY PART: Zygomatic Arches

POSITION/PROJECTION: Tangential—May Method

ANATOMY: A tangential projection of the zygomatic arch free of superimposed shadows. It is used for persons with flat cheekbones or depressed fractures.

PATIENT/PART POSITION: With the patient's head resting on the fully extended chin, place the infraorbitomeatal line as parallel as possible to the image receptor. Rotate the patient's head 15 degrees away from the side being examined. Center the image receptor to coincide with a point 3 inches distal to the most prominent point of the zygoma.

CENTRAL RAY LOCATION/ANGLE: The central ray is directed perpendicular to the infraorbitomeatal line approximately 1½ inches posterior to the outer canthus.

NOTES:

MANDIBLE

GENERAL TECHNICAL TIPS:
DID YOU
REMEMBER TO?

■ properly identify the patient?

■ properly shield the patient?

■ collimate to the part?

■ use an extension cone, if available?

■ use a small focal spot?

■ perform the axiolaterals with the patient in a sitting or standing position, if possible?

BODY PART: Mandible

POSITION/PROJECTION: Posteroanterior—Body

ANATOMY: A posteroanterior projection of the mandibular body.

PATIENT/PART POSITION: Place the patient in the prone position. Rest the patient's head on the nose and chin. Center the image receptor at the level of the lips. The midsagittal plane of the head is perpendicular to the plane of the image receptor.

CENTRAL RAY LOCATION/ANGLE: The central ray is directed perpendicular to the midpoint of the image receptor.

NOTES:

BODY PART: Mandible

POSITION/PROJECTION: Axial—Rami

ANATOMY: The mandibular rami and temporomandibular joints in a posteroanterior projection.

PATIENT/PART POSITION: The patient is prone, with the head resting on the nose and chin. Center the image receptor at the tip of the nose and place the midsagittal plane perpendicular to the image receptor.

CENTRAL RAY LOCATION/ANGLE: The central ray is directed midway between the temporomandibular joints at an angle of 30 degrees cephalad.

NOTES:

BODY PART: Mandible

POSITION/PROJECTION: Axiolateral

ANATOMY: An axiolateral projection of the mandible. The half of the mandible nearest the image receptor is best demonstrated.

PATIENT/PART POSITION: With the patient semiprone, adjust the image receptor under the cheek, extending the head and neck and rotating the patient's face towards the table, so that the long axis of the mandibular body is parallel with the plane of the image receptor.

CENTRAL RAY LOCATION/ANGLE: The central ray is directed to the midpoint of the image receptor at an angle of 25 degrees cephalad.

NOTES:

TEMPOROMANDIBULAR JOINTS

GENERAL TECHNICAL TIPS:
DID YOU
REMEMBER TO?

- ■ properly identify the patient?
- ■ properly shield the patient?
- ■ collimate to the part?
- ■ use an extension cone, if available?
- ■ use a small focal spot?
- ■ do both sides and correctly mark each film?
- ■ do each side in both open and closed mouth positions?

BODY PART: Temporomandibular Joints

POSITION/PROJECTION: Lateral Transcranial

ANATOMY: The temporomandibular joints in the open and closed positions.

PATIENT/PART POSITION: The patient is in a semiprone position. Rotate the patient's head towards the table so that the head is resting on the cheek. Center at a point ½ inch anterior to the dependent external auditory meatus. The acanthiomeatal line is parallel to the image receptor.

CENTRAL RAY LOCATION/ANGLE: The central ray is directed to the midpoint of the image receptor at a 15-degree caudal angle. It will exit at the dependent temporomandibular joint.

NOTES:

BODY PART: Temporomandibular Joints

POSITION/PROJECTION: Axial Transcranial

ANATOMY: The temporomandibular joints in the open and closed positions.

PATIENT/PART POSITION: Place the patient's head in a true lateral skull position. Adjust the patient's head so that the midsagittal plane is parallel with, and the interpupillary line perpendicular to, the table or upright Bucky. Center at a point ½ inch anterior to and 1 inch below the dependent external auditory meatus.

CENTRAL RAY LOCATION/ANGLE: The central ray is directed to the midpoint of the image receptor at a 25- to 30-degree caudal angle, entering the upper parietal region and exiting at the dependent temporomandibular joint.

NOTES:

PARANASAL SINUSES

GENERAL TECHNICAL TIPS:
DID YOU
REMEMBER TO?

- ■ properly identify the patient?
- ■ properly shield the patient?
- ■ collimate to the part?
- ■ use an extension cone, if available?
- ■ use a small focal spot?
- ■ do all views erect, if possible?
- ■ place the mentomeatal line perpendicular for a Waters method position?
- ■ check that the interpupillary line is perpendicular in the lateral?
- ■ perform the Schuller method position with the patient in a sitting or standing position?
- ■ check your source-to-image distance?

BODY PART: Paranasal Sinuses

POSITION/PROJECTION: Posteroanterior—Modified Caldwell Method

ANATOMY: The frontal sinuses and anterior ethmoid air cells.

PATIENT/PART POSITION: The patient is placed prone on the table or facing the upright grid device with the forehead and nose placed against the table or upright Bucky. The midsagittal and orbitomeatal lines are placed perpendicular to the image receptor. The top of the image receptor is placed 1½ inches above the vertex.

CENTRAL RAY LOCATION/ANGLE: The central ray is directed 15 degrees caudally to pass through the nasion.

NOTES:

In the original Caldwell method, the central ray is directed to the glabella at a caudal angle of 23 degrees to the glabellomeatal line.

BODY PART: Paranasal Sinuses

POSITION/PROJECTION: Parietoacanthial—Waters Method

TUBE

ANATOMY: An unobstructed frontal projection of the maxillary sinuses above the petrous pyramids.

PATIENT/PART POSITION: Center the midsagittal plane of the patient's head to the midline of the table, resting the head on the tip of the extended chin. The midsagittal plane is perpendicular to the image receptor. Adjust the flexion of the head so that the orbitomeatal line forms an angle of 37 degrees with the plane of the image receptor.

CENTRAL RAY LOCATION/ANGLE: The central ray is directed perpendicular to the image receptor to exit at the acanthion.

TUBE

NOTES:

BODY PART: Paranasal Sinuses

POSITION/PROJECTION: Lateral

ANATOMY: A lateral projection of the anteroposterior and superior inferior dimensions of the paranasal sinuses.

PATIENT/PART POSITION: Place the patient in a lateral skull position. Center the outer canthus to the midpoint of the table or upright Bucky.

CENTRAL RAY LOCATION/ANGLE: The central ray is directed perpendicular to the midpoint of the image receptor.

NOTES:

BODY PART: Paranasal Sinuses

POSITION/PROJECTION: Submentovertical—Schuller Method

ANATOMY: An axial projection of the sphenoid sinuses, the posterior ethmoid cells, the antra, and the nasal fossae.

PATIENT/PART POSITION: The patient is either sitting, with the vertex resting against the upright Bucky, or supine on the table with pillows or sponges under the shoulders to assist in hyperextending the head and neck. The infraorbitomeatal line is adjusted as parallel as possible to the image receptor. The vertex of the head is rested on the table and the midsagittal plane is adjusted so that it is perpendicular to the image receptor.

CENTRAL RAY LOCATION/ANGLE: The central ray is directed perpendicular to the infraorbitomeatal line entering midway between the mandibular angles. The degree of angulation of the central ray depends on the degree of hyperextension of the patient's head and neck.

NOTES:

TEMPORAL BONE—MASTOIDS

GENERAL TECHNICAL TIPS:
DID YOU
REMEMBER TO?

- properly identify the patient?
- properly shield the patient?
- collimate to the part?
- use an extension cone, if available?
- use a small focal spot?
- do both sides and correctly mark each film?
- center the side that's down in the Law, Henschen, Lysholm, and Schuller method positions?
- center the side away from the film in the Hickey method position?
- check your source-to-image distance?

BODY PART: Temporal Bone—Mastoids

POSITION/PROJECTION: Axiolateral—Modified Law Method

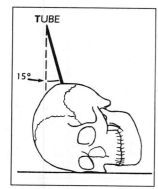

ANATOMY: A lateral transcranial projection of the mastoid air cells, and the superimposed internal and external auditory meati.

PATIENT/PART POSITION: Center the image receptor to a point 1 inch posterior to the dependent external auditory meatus and adjust the head so that the infraorbitomeatal line is parallel with the plane of the image receptor. The interpupillary line should be perpendicular to the image receptor. The midsagittal plane of the skull is rotated 15 degrees toward the table or upright Bucky.

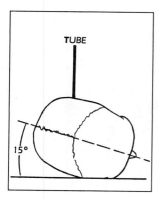

CENTRAL RAY LOCATION/ANGLE: The central ray is directed to the midpoint of the image receptor at a caudal angle of 15 degrees.

NOTES:

BODY PART: Temporal Bone—Mastoids

POSITION/PROJECTION: Anteroposterior Tangential—Hickey Method

ANATOMY: An anteroposterior tangential projection of the mastoid process projected free of adjacent bony structures.

PATIENT/PART POSITION: Tape the auricles forward. The patient is either supine on the table or in an anteroposterior position at an upright Bucky. Center the midsagittal plane and rotate it away from the side being examined until it forms a 55-degree angle with the plane of the table or upright Bucky. Place the infraorbitomeatal line perpendicular to the image receptor and center the image receptor 1 inch below the palpable tip of the mastoid process.

CENTRAL RAY LOCATION/ANGLE: The central ray is directed at a 15-degree caudal angle to the midpoint of the image receptor.

NOTES:

BODY PART: Temporal Bone—Mastoids

POSITION/PROJECTION: Axiolateral—Henschen, Schuller, and Lysholm Methods

ANATOMY: An axiolateral projection of the following:

a. Henschen—the mastoid cells, the internal and external auditory meati.

b. Schuller—pneumatic structure of the mastoid process, the internal and external auditory meati, the sinus, and the dural plates.

c. Lysholm—the mastoid air cells, the labyrinth area, the external auditory meatus, and the carotid canal.

PATIENT/PART POSITION: The patient's head is rested in a true lateral position. Center to a point ¾ inch inferior to the dependent mastoid process for the Schuller and Lysholm methods. Center to the dependent mastoid for the Henschen method.

CENTRAL RAY LOCATION/ANGLE: The central ray is directed through the dependent external auditory meatus at the following angle(s):

a. Henschen: 15 degrees caudal.

b. Schuller: 25 degrees caudal.

c. Lysholm: 35 degrees caudal.

NOTES:

TEMPORAL BONE—PETROUS PORTION

GENERAL TECHNICAL TIPS: DID YOU REMEMBER TO?

- properly identify the patient?
- properly shield the patient?
- collimate to the part?
- use an extension cone, if available?
- use a small focal spot?
- do both sides and correctly mark each film?
- center the side that's down in the Stenvers method position?
- center the side that's up in the Arcelin method position?
- check your source-to-image distance?

BODY PART: Temporal Bone—Petrous Portion

POSITION/PROJECTION: Submentovertical—Schuller Method

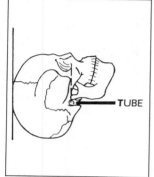

ANATOMY: A full basal projection of the cranium, including the petrous pyramids, the mastoid processes, the foramina ovale and spinosum, the carotid canals, the sphenoid and maxillary sinuses, the mandible, the foramen magnum, the odontoid process and the entire atlas.

PATIENT/PART POSITION: The patient is either sitting, with the vertex resting against the upright Bucky, or supine on the table with pillows or sponges under the shoulders to assist in hyperextending the head and neck. The infraorbitomeatal line is adjusted as parallel as possible to the image receptor. The vertex of the head is rested on the table or on the upright Bucky and midsagittal plane adjusted so that it is perpendicular to the image receptor.

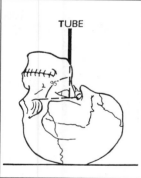

CENTRAL RAY LOCATION/ANGLE: The central ray is directed perpendicular to the infraorbitomeatal line, passing through the sella turcica. The degree of angulation of the central ray will depend on the degree of hyperextension of the patient's head and neck.

NOTES:

BODY PART: Temporal Bone—Petrous Portion

POSITION/PROJECTION: AP Axial—Grashey Method

ANATOMY: An AP axial projection of the occipital region, the bilateral petrous pyramids, the foramen magnum, the internal auditory canals, and the labyrinths. The dorsum sellae and posterior clinoids are demonstrated within the shadow of the foramen magnum.

PATIENT/PART POSITION: The patient is either supine on the table or with the back against an upright Bucky. The midsagittal and orbitomeatal lines are placed perpendicular to the image receptor.*

CENTRAL RAY LOCATION/ANGLE: The central ray is directed caudally to pass through the foramen magnum at a 30-degree angle.
*Some patients may require that the infraorbitomeatal line be placed perpendicular to the image receptor. In these cases, a 37-degree caudal angle will be used.

NOTES:

BODY PART: Temporal Bone—Petrous Portion

POSITION/PROJECTION: Posterior Profile—Stenvers Method

ANATOMY: A posterior profile projection of the pars petrosa projected parallel to the image receptor. Structures include the mastoid process, internal auditory canal, and bony labyrinth.

PATIENT/PART POSITION: Center a point 1 inch anterior to the external auditory meatus to the center of the table or upright Bucky. Rest the head on the forehead, nose, and zygoma. The midsagittal plane should form an angle of 45 degrees with the plane of the image receptor. Adjust the flexion of the head and neck so that the infraorbitomeatal line is perpendicular to the image receptor.

CENTRAL RAY LOCATION/ANGLE: The central ray is directed to the midpoint of the image receptor at a cephalic angle of 12 degrees.

NOTES:

BODY PART: Temporal Bone—Petrous Portion

POSITION/PROJECTION: Anterior Profile—Arcelin Method

ANATOMY: An anterior profile projection of the petrous portion of the temporal bone (exact opposite of a Stenvers).

PATIENT/PART POSITION: The patient is in either a supine position or AP to an upright Bucky. Rotate the patient's head approximately 45 degrees away from the side being examined and center at a point 1 inch anterior to the external auditory meatus. Adjust the flexion of the head and neck so that the infraorbitomeatal line is perpendicular to the image receptor.

CENTRAL RAY LOCATION/ANGLE: The central ray is directed 10 degrees caudad to the midpoint of the image receptor.

NOTES:

BIBLIOGRAPHY

Anderson, K. N., and Anderson, L. E. (1990). *Mosby's Pocket Dictionary of Medicine, Nursing, and Allied Health.* St. Louis: Mosby–Year Book.

Ballinger, P. W. (1992). *Pocket Guide to Radiography*, 2nd ed. St. Louis: Mosby–Year Book.

——. (1991). *Merrill's Atlas of Radiologic Positions and Radiologic Procedures*, 7th ed. St. Louis: Mosby–Year Book.

Bontrager, K., and Anthony, B. T. (1987). *Textbook of Radiographic Positioning and Related Anatomy*, 2nd ed. Denver: Multi-Media.

Donohue, D. P. (1984). *An Analysis of Radiographic Quality.* Rockville, Maryland: Aspen Systems.

Drafke, M. (1990). *Trauma and Mobile Radiography.* Philadelphia: F. A. Davis.

Ehrlich, R. A., and Givens, E. M. (1989). *Patient Care in Radiography*, 3rd ed. St. Louis: Mosby–Year Book.

Eisenberg, R. L., Dennis, C., and May, C. (1989). *Radiographic Positioning.* Boston: Little, Brown & Co.

Gurley, L. T., and Callaway, W. J. (1986). *Introduction to Radiologic Technology*, 2nd ed. St. Louis: Mosby–Year Book.

Mace, J. D., and Kowalczyk, N. (1988). *Radiographic Pathology for Technologists.* St. Louis: Mosby–Year Book.

Rambo, B. J., and Wood, L. A. (1982). *Nursing Skills for Clinical Practice*, 3rd ed. Philadelphia: W. B. Saunders.

Swallow, R. A., and Naylor, E. (1986). *Clark's Positioning in Radiography*, 11th ed. Rockville, Maryland: Aspen Systems.

Thompson, T. T. (1979). *Cahoon's Formulating X-Ray Techniques*, 9th ed. Durham, North Carolina: Duke University Press.

Torres, L. (1989). *Basic Medical Techniques and Patient Care for Radiologic Technologists*, 3rd ed. Philadelphia: J. B. Lippincott.

Tortora, G., and Anagnostakos, N. (1990). *Principles of Anatomy and Physiology*, 6th ed. New York: Harper Collins.

Wicke, L. (1987). *Atlas of Radiologic Anatomy*, 4th ed. Baltimore: Urban and Schwarzenberg.

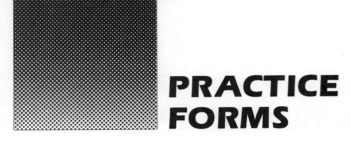

PRACTICE FORMS

Blank practice forms are provided here. Their use is described in the note to the student on page x.

BODY PART:

_____

_____

POSITION/PROJECTION:

_____

_____

ANATOMY:

_____

_____

_____

PATIENT/PART POSITION:

_____

_____

_____

_____

CENTRAL RAY LOCATION/ANGLE:

_____

_____

NOTES:

_____

_____

_____

_____

_____

_____

_____

_____

_____

_____

NOTES CON'T.

BODY PART:

POSITION/PROJECTION:

ANATOMY:

PATIENT/PART POSITION:

CENTRAL RAY LOCATION/ANGLE:

NOTES:

NOTES CON'T.

BODY PART:

_____

_____

_____

POSITION/PROJECTION:

_____

_____

_____

ANATOMY:

_____

_____

_____

_____

PATIENT/PART POSITION:

_____

_____

_____

_____

_____

_____

CENTRAL RAY LOCATION/ANGLE:

_____

_____

_____

NOTES:

_____

_____

_____

_____

_____

_____

_____

_____

_____

_____

NOTES CON'T.

BODY PART:

_____

_____

_____

POSITION/PROJECTION:

_____

_____

_____

ANATOMY:

_____

_____

_____

_____

PATIENT/PART POSITION:

_____

_____

_____

_____

_____

_____

CENTRAL RAY LOCATION/ANGLE:

_____

_____

_____

NOTES:

_____

_____

_____

_____

_____

_____

_____

_____

_____

_____

_____

_____

NOTES CON'T.

BODY PART:

_____

_____

_____

POSITION/PROJECTION:

_____

_____

_____

ANATOMY:

_____

_____

_____

_____

PATIENT/PART POSITION:

_____

_____

_____

_____

_____

CENTRAL RAY LOCATION/ANGLE:

_____

_____

_____

NOTES:

_____

_____

_____

_____

_____

_____

_____

_____

_____

_____

_____

NOTES CON'T.

BODY PART:

_____
_____
_____

POSITION/PROJECTION:

_____
_____
_____

ANATOMY:

_____
_____
_____
_____

PATIENT/PART POSITION:

_____
_____
_____
_____
_____

CENTRAL RAY LOCATION/ANGLE:

_____
_____
_____

NOTES:

_____
_____
_____
_____
_____
_____
_____
_____
_____
_____

NOTES CON'T.

BODY PART:

_____

_____

POSITION/PROJECTION:

_____

_____

ANATOMY:

_____

_____

_____

_____

PATIENT/PART POSITION:

_____

_____

_____

_____

_____

CENTRAL RAY LOCATION/ANGLE:

_____

_____

NOTES:

_____

_____

_____

_____

_____

_____

_____

_____

_____

_____

_____

NOTES CON'T.

BODY PART:

_____

_____

_____

POSITION/PROJECTION:

_____

_____

_____

ANATOMY:

_____

_____

_____

_____

PATIENT/PART POSITION:

_____

_____

_____

_____

_____

CENTRAL RAY LOCATION/ANGLE:

_____

_____

_____

NOTES:

_____

_____

_____

_____

_____

_____

_____

_____

_____

_____

_____

NOTES CON'T.

BODY PART:

_____

_____

_____

POSITION/PROJECTION:

_____

_____

_____

ANATOMY:

_____

_____

_____

_____

PATIENT/PART POSITION:

_____

_____

_____

_____

_____

_____

CENTRAL RAY LOCATION/ANGLE:

_____

_____

_____

NOTES:

_____

_____

_____

_____

_____

_____

_____

_____

_____

_____

_____

_____

_____

NOTES CON'T.

BODY PART:

POSITION/PROJECTION:

ANATOMY:

PATIENT/PART POSITION:

CENTRAL RAY LOCATION/ANGLE:

NOTES:

NOTES CON'T.

BODY PART:

_____

_____

_____

POSITION/PROJECTION:

_____

_____

_____

ANATOMY:

_____

_____

_____

_____

PATIENT/PART POSITION:

_____

_____

_____

_____

_____

_____

CENTRAL RAY LOCATION/ANGLE:

_____

_____

_____

NOTES:

_____

_____

_____

_____

_____

_____

_____

_____

_____

_____

_____

_____

NOTES CON'T.

BODY PART:

_____

_____

POSITION/PROJECTION:

_____

_____

ANATOMY:

_____

_____

_____

PATIENT/PART POSITION:

_____

_____

_____

_____

CENTRAL RAY LOCATION/ANGLE:

_____

_____

NOTES:

_____

_____

_____

_____

_____

_____

_____

_____

_____

_____

_____

NOTES CON'T.

BODY PART:

_____

_____

POSITION/PROJECTION:

_____

_____

ANATOMY:

_____

_____

_____

PATIENT/PART POSITION:

_____

_____

_____

_____

_____

CENTRAL RAY LOCATION/ANGLE:

_____

_____

NOTES:

_____

_____

_____

_____

_____

_____

_____

_____

_____

_____

_____

NOTES CON'T.

BODY PART:

_____

_____

POSITION/PROJECTION:

_____

_____

ANATOMY:

_____

_____

_____

PATIENT/PART POSITION:

_____

_____

_____

_____

_____

CENTRAL RAY LOCATION/ANGLE:

_____

_____

_____

NOTES:

_____

_____

_____

_____

_____

_____

_____

_____

_____

_____

NOTES CON'T.

BODY PART:

_____
_____
_____

POSITION/PROJECTION:

_____
_____
_____

ANATOMY:

_____
_____
_____
_____

PATIENT/PART POSITION:

_____
_____
_____
_____
_____
_____

CENTRAL RAY LOCATION/ANGLE:

_____
_____
_____

NOTES:

_____
_____
_____
_____
_____
_____
_____
_____
_____
_____
_____
_____

NOTES CON'T.

BODY PART:

_____
_____
_____

POSITION/PROJECTION:

_____
_____
_____

ANATOMY:

_____
_____
_____
_____

PATIENT/PART POSITION:

_____
_____
_____
_____
_____
_____

CENTRAL RAY LOCATION/ANGLE:

_____
_____
_____

NOTES:

_____
_____
_____
_____
_____
_____
_____
_____
_____
_____

NOTES CON'T.

BODY PART:

_____
_____
_____

POSITION/PROJECTION:

_____
_____
_____

ANATOMY:

_____
_____
_____
_____

PATIENT/PART POSITION:

_____
_____
_____
_____
_____
_____

CENTRAL RAY LOCATION/ANGLE:

_____
_____
_____

NOTES:

_____
_____
_____
_____
_____
_____
_____
_____
_____
_____
_____

NOTES CON'T.

BODY PART:

_____
_____
_____

POSITION/PROJECTION:

_____
_____
_____

ANATOMY:

_____
_____
_____
_____

PATIENT/PART POSITION:

_____
_____
_____
_____
_____
_____

CENTRAL RAY LOCATION/ANGLE:

_____
_____
_____

NOTES:

_____
_____
_____
_____
_____
_____
_____
_____
_____
_____
_____

NOTES CON'T.

BODY PART:

_____

_____

_____

POSITION/PROJECTION:

_____

_____

_____

ANATOMY:

_____

_____

_____

_____

PATIENT/PART POSITION:

_____

_____

_____

_____

_____

CENTRAL RAY LOCATION/ANGLE:

_____

_____

_____

NOTES:

_____

_____

_____

_____

_____

_____

_____

_____

_____

_____

_____

NOTES CON'T.

BODY PART:

_____

_____

_____

POSITION/PROJECTION:

_____

_____

ANATOMY:

_____

_____

_____

_____

PATIENT/PART POSITION:

_____

_____

_____

_____

_____

CENTRAL RAY LOCATION/ANGLE:

_____

_____

_____

NOTES:

_____

_____

_____

_____

_____

_____

_____

_____

_____

_____

_____

NOTES CON'T.

BODY PART:

POSITION/PROJECTION:

ANATOMY:

PATIENT/PART POSITION:

CENTRAL RAY LOCATION/ANGLE:

NOTES:

NOTES CON'T.

BODY PART:

_____
_____
_____

POSITION/PROJECTION:

_____
_____
_____

ANATOMY:

_____
_____
_____
_____

PATIENT/PART POSITION:

_____
_____
_____
_____
_____
_____

CENTRAL RAY LOCATION/ANGLE:

_____
_____
_____

NOTES:

_____
_____
_____
_____
_____
_____
_____
_____
_____
_____
_____
_____

NOTES CON'T.

BODY PART:

_____
_____
_____

POSITION/PROJECTION:

_____
_____
_____

ANATOMY:

_____
_____
_____
_____

PATIENT/PART POSITION:

_____
_____
_____
_____
_____

CENTRAL RAY LOCATION/ANGLE:

_____
_____
_____

NOTES:

_____
_____
_____
_____
_____
_____
_____
_____
_____
_____
_____

NOTES CON'T.

BODY PART:

POSITION/PROJECTION:

ANATOMY:

PATIENT/PART POSITION:

CENTRAL RAY LOCATION/ANGLE:

NOTES:

NOTES CON'T.

BODY PART:

_____

_____

POSITION/PROJECTION:

_____

_____

ANATOMY:

_____

_____

_____

PATIENT/PART POSITION:

_____

_____

_____

_____

CENTRAL RAY LOCATION/ANGLE:

_____

_____

NOTES:

_____

_____

_____

_____

_____

_____

_____

_____

_____

_____

NOTES CON'T.

BODY PART:

_____

_____

_____

POSITION/PROJECTION:

_____

_____

_____

ANATOMY:

_____

_____

_____

_____

PATIENT/PART POSITION:

_____

_____

_____

_____

_____

CENTRAL RAY LOCATION/ANGLE:

_____

_____

_____

NOTES:

_____

_____

_____

_____

_____

_____

_____

_____

_____

_____

_____

NOTES CON'T.

BODY PART: _____

_____

_____

POSITION/PROJECTION: _____

_____

_____

ANATOMY: _____

_____

_____

_____

PATIENT/PART POSITION: _____

_____

_____

_____

_____

_____

CENTRAL RAY LOCATION/ANGLE: _____

_____

_____

NOTES: _____

_____

_____

_____

_____

_____

_____

_____

_____

_____

_____

_____

NOTES CON'T.

BODY PART:

POSITION/PROJECTION:

ANATOMY:

PATIENT/PART POSITION:

CENTRAL RAY LOCATION/ANGLE:

NOTES:

NOTES CON'T.

BODY PART:

_____
_____
_____

POSITION/PROJECTION:

_____
_____
_____

ANATOMY:

_____
_____
_____
_____

PATIENT/PART POSITION:

_____
_____
_____
_____
_____
_____

CENTRAL RAY LOCATION/ANGLE:

_____
_____
_____

NOTES:

_____
_____
_____
_____
_____
_____
_____
_____
_____
_____
_____
_____

NOTES CON'T.

BODY PART:

_____
_____
_____

POSITION/PROJECTION:

_____
_____
_____

ANATOMY:

_____
_____
_____
_____

PATIENT/PART POSITION:

_____
_____
_____
_____
_____

CENTRAL RAY LOCATION/ANGLE:

_____
_____
_____

NOTES:

_____
_____
_____
_____
_____
_____
_____
_____
_____
_____

NOTES CON'T.

BODY PART:

_____

_____

POSITION/PROJECTION:

_____

_____

ANATOMY:

_____

_____

_____

PATIENT/PART POSITION:

_____

_____

_____

_____

_____

CENTRAL RAY LOCATION/ANGLE:

_____

_____

NOTES:

_____

_____

_____

_____

_____

_____

_____

_____

_____

_____

NOTES CON'T.

BODY PART:

_____

_____

_____

POSITION/PROJECTION:

_____

_____

_____

ANATOMY:

_____

_____

_____

_____

PATIENT/PART POSITION:

_____

_____

_____

_____

_____

CENTRAL RAY LOCATION/ANGLE:

_____

_____

_____

NOTES:

_____

_____

_____

_____

_____

_____

_____

_____

_____

_____

_____

NOTES CON'T.

BODY PART:

_____

_____

_____

POSITION/PROJECTION:

_____

_____

_____

ANATOMY:

_____

_____

_____

_____

PATIENT/PART POSITION:

_____

_____

_____

_____

_____

_____

CENTRAL RAY LOCATION/ANGLE:

_____

_____

_____

NOTES:

_____

_____

_____

_____

_____

_____

_____

_____

_____

_____

_____

NOTES CON'T.

BODY PART:

POSITION/PROJECTION:

ANATOMY:

PATIENT/PART POSITION:

CENTRAL RAY LOCATION/ANGLE:

NOTES:

NOTES CON'T.

BODY PART:

_____
_____
_____

POSITION/PROJECTION:

_____
_____

ANATOMY:

_____
_____
_____
_____

PATIENT/PART POSITION:

_____
_____
_____
_____
_____

CENTRAL RAY LOCATION/ANGLE:

_____
_____
_____

NOTES:

_____
_____
_____
_____
_____
_____
_____
_____
_____
_____
_____
_____

NOTES CON'T.

BODY PART:

_____

_____

POSITION/PROJECTION:

_____

_____

ANATOMY:

_____

_____

_____

PATIENT/PART POSITION:

_____

_____

_____

_____

_____

CENTRAL RAY LOCATION/ANGLE:

_____

_____

NOTES:

_____

_____

_____

_____

_____

_____

_____

_____

_____

_____

NOTES CON'T.

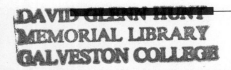